Praise for
MATT FITZGERALD

"Extremely well done . . . A must for marathoners!"
— *Library Journal*

"Basically it's the *The 7 Habits of Highly Effective People* for the cycling set, and it's a great read."
— *Bicycling*

"Being a three-time Olympian, I thought I knew all there was to know about diet and training, but Matt blew me away. I can't wait to start implementing all his knowledge into my running."
— SHALANE FLANAGAN, Olympic bronze medalist and
    American record-holder

"This book teaches you how to avoid the many pitfalls of fueling for endurance running and how to use nutrition to improve your performance. I wouldn't marathon without it."
— JENNY HADFIELD, author of *Marathoning for Mortals*

"Fitzgerald is a fountain of information on current research studies and findings from the sciences of healthy nutrition and exercise performance."
— *Ultrarunning Magazine*

"[Fitzgerald's] perspective on hotly contested topics in sports science is always well-informed, practical, and leavened with enough skepticism to avoid jumping on and off every passing bandwagon. . . . He's entirely reasonable in differentiating between proven 'you must do this' tactics, and more speculative 'experiment with this if you're interested' tactics. . . . A nice intro to endurance nutrition."

—RunnersWorld.com

"If you're looking to get to your peak performance weight or explore the mind-body connection of running, writer Matt Fitzgerald has some advice for you. . . . Fitzgerald, an expert in endurance training and nutrition, explores a wide range of topics and cutting-edge developments from the world of running and endurance sports."

—ESPN.com

"In his latest book, Matt Fitzgerald successfully explains the mind-body method of running. . . . Anyone trying to improve and realize their true running potential should read *Run*."

—KARA GOUCHER, 2008 Olympian and world championship medalist

"To be a great athlete, you need more than natural ability; you need mental strength to keep going when your body wants to quit. In his new book, writer Matt Fitzgerald dives into the research behind these coping skills and highlights the top athletes who use them. Anyone, whether pro or everyday exercisers, can use these tactics to push further."

—*Men's Journal*

"Fitzgerald is going to go down as one of the most competent and prolific authors of books for serious runners covering just about every legitimate aspect of the all-important runner's lifestyle."

—LetsRun.com

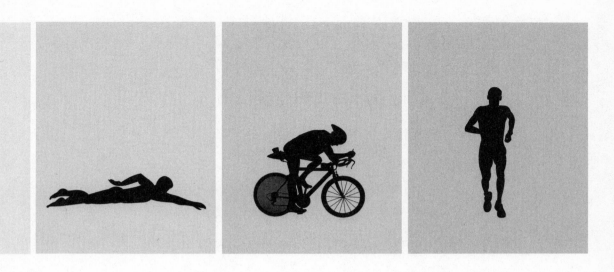

80/20 TRIATHLON

Also by Matt Fitzgerald

The Endurance Diet

How Bad Do You Want It?

Iron War

The New Rules of Marathon and Half-Marathon Nutrition

80/20 Running

Racing Weight Cookbook

Racing Weight

Brain Training for Runners

Performance Nutrition for Runners

80/20 TRIATHLON

Discover the
Breakthrough Elite-Training Formula
for Ultimate Fitness and
Performance at All Levels

—

MATT FITZGERALD
DAVID WARDEN

Da Capo

LIFE
LONG

Copyright © 2018 by Matt Fitzgerald and David Warden

Photographs by Sarah Cotton

Hachette Book Group supports the right to free expression and the value of copyright. The purpose of copyright is to encourage writers and artists to produce the creative works that enrich our culture.

The scanning, uploading, and distribution of this book without permission is a theft of the author's intellectual property. If you would like permission to use material from the book (other than for review purposes), please contact permissions@hbgusa.com. Thank you for your support of the author's rights.

Da Capo Press
Hachette Book Group
1290 Avenue of the Americas, New York, NY 10104
www.dacapopress.com
@DaCapoPress

Printed in the United States of America

First Edition: September 2018

Published by Da Capo Press, an imprint of Perseus Books, LLC, a subsidiary of Hachette Book Group, Inc. The Da Capo Press name and logo is a trademark of the Hachette Book Group.

The Hachette Speakers Bureau provides a wide range of authors for speaking events. To find out more, go to www.hachettespeakersbureau.com or call (866) 376-6591.

The publisher is not responsible for websites (or their content) that are not owned by the publisher.

Print book interior design by Cynthia Young at Sagecraft

Library of Congress Cataloging-in-Publication Data has been applied for.
ISBNs: 978-0-7382-3468-7 (paperback), 978-0-7382-3469-4 (ebook)

LSC-C

10 9 8 7 6 5 4 3 2 1

CONTENTS

FOREWORD

by

DR. STEPHEN SEILER
Professor in Sport Science
University of Agder,
Kristiansand, Norway

I love laboratories. When I was eleven years old, my parents gave me the small walk-in closet under the stairs to create my first laboratory. I had lots of chemistry equipment, a microscope, and other science gear to play with when I returned home from school, where, to be honest, sports were my favorite activity. Ever since then I have been consumed by two interests: sports and science. Lucky for me, my two passions came together in the form of sport science, and I have spent many, many hours in laboratories since those days under the stairs. The labs have grown, with room for students, treadmills, bicycle ergometers, and advanced measurement devices, all designed to help us study the physiology, biomechanics, and psychology of training and performance.

Yet the largest and most powerful sport science *laboratory* on the planet has no white lab coats hanging on the wall. It has no walls. This laboratory is on forest trails, in lakes and pools, and on the asphalt roads where tens of thousands of athletes *labor* daily with one goal in mind: to get from point A to point B as fast as possible. Training that works is retained and passed on to others, and training that does not is ultimately discarded.

My 80/20 intensity distribution model that I presented for the sport science community about 15 years ago was developed in *that* global laboratory by the best endurance athletes in the world over many decades. Since then, my lab and the labs of many others have carefully studied different aspects of training intensity distribution, creating a *scientist laboratory/athlete laboratory* feedback loop. I have spent my career attempting to operate at this intersection between science and practice. But translating science into practice remains hard, and we scientists are not often very good at it. I hate to admit it, but Matt Fitzgerald has translated my own research findings into daily practice guidelines far better than I could myself.

First with *80/20 Running* and now with *80/20 Triathlon*, Matt has used his experience as athlete, coach, and writer to merge all the findings from these two laboratory settings into a thoughtful, honest recipe book for triathletes of all levels. The science is here, embedded in every page. But it is the practical "nuts and bolts" aspect that makes the difference, offering sorely needed guidance in the challenging process of designing and executing a training plan that is understandable, flexible, and sustainable.

In no endurance sport is the training process more complex than in triathlon. My most challenging questions seem to come when I give lectures where triathlon coaches and athletes are in the audience. Long-term planning for a runner, a swimmer, or a cyclist is demanding enough. Putting all three together is a nightmare for scientists who like to focus on one variable at a time. Triathlon training and performance will continue to be a topic of research in the years to come. But we already know that the 80/20 method works in all endurance sports, including triathlon. And it works whether you train four times a week or fourteen. This book provides sensible plans for triathletes across this spectrum. These plans will reduce your uncertainty and greatly increase the likelihood that you will reach your goals. At the same time, each reader is a laboratory of one, experimenting, observing, and adjusting. I am convinced that *80/20 Triathlon* will create a sound, sustainable platform for your own fascinating training adventure. You are all athlete scientists. Enjoy your countless hours in the greatest laboratory on the planet!

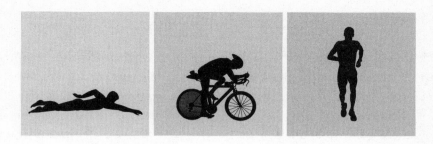

1

The Most Effective Way to Train

Let's begin with a thought experiment. Suppose you trained for your next triathlon (or your first triathlon, as the case may be) by chopping wood for 30 minutes every morning. Do you think you would perform better or worse on race day than you would if you trained the way you normally do? The answer is obvious: worse.

Now let's suppose that you trained for your next triathlon (or your first) by reducing the amount of time you spend swimming, cycling, and running each week by 75 percent. How would this affect your performance? Again, negatively.

Finally, imagine training for a triathlon by doing all of your swimming, cycling, and running at top speed. Same question: Would this approach produce better or worse race results than the way you currently train? Same answer: worse.

The point we're trying to make with these hypothetical scenarios is that some ways of training for triathlons are more effective than other ways. The first example concerns the principle of *specificity*. To be effective, the training you do must be specific to the thing you're training for. It goes without saying (but we'll say it anyway) that swimming, cycling, and running are considerably more triathlon-specific than chopping wood is.

The second example relates to training *volume*, or the amount of training you do. To get the best results from your training, you need to hit the sweet spot between too little and too much. Of course, the volume of training that is optimal for each individual triathlete depends on experience and other factors, but a sudden three-quarters reduction of training volume won't help any triathlete except one who's currently training way too much.

The last of the three hypothetical scenarios we offered concerns another important training variable: *intensity*, or how hard you swim, bike, and run relative to your personal limits. Whatever the most effective way of manipulating this variable may be (and we won't leave this question unanswered for very long), it most certainly isn't full speed all the time.

It follows from the fact that some ways of training are more effective than others that there must exist an *optimal* way to train: a set of methods encompassing specificity, volume, intensity, and other factors that is more effective than any alternative. While individual considerations, such as experience, certainly influence each athlete's optimal way to train, to the extent that we're all human, there has to be an overall approach to training that works best for everyone. So, then: What is the most effective way to train for the sport of triathlon?

The 80/20 Rule

Only recently has science made significant progress in identifying universal best practices in endurance training. The leading researcher in this area is Stephen Seiler, an American exercise physiologist based in Norway. In the early 2000s, Seiler made what is perhaps the most important discovery in the history of endurance sports science: the 80/20 Rule. Through rigorous analysis of the training methods used by elite endurance athletes in a variety of endurance disciplines, he found that world-class cyclists, runners, triathletes, and others do approximately 80 percent of their training at low intensity and the remaining 20 percent at moderate and high intensities. But they didn't always. Historical records that Seiler reviewed indicate that elite endurance athletes of past generations trained very differently than today's do. This fact, when considered alongside the fact that today's top endurance athletes are much faster than their predecessors, led Seiler to conclude that a long-term process of trial and error had gradually exposed the training methods that produced the best results, and that the 80/20 Rule was the cornerstone of the optimal way to train for endurance performance.

The obvious next step was to determine whether the methods that appeared to work best for world-class athletes were optimal for recreational endurance athletes as well. Carefully designed studies have revealed that they are indeed. Everyday athletes who work out as little as 45 minutes a day have been shown to improve more when following the 80/20 Rule than when they train with greater intensity.

These findings would be scarcely worth a shrug if most nonelite athletes followed the 80/20 Rule already. But they don't. The typical age-group triathlete does less than 70 percent of his or her training at low intensity, and many do a lot less. Instead of spending 48 minutes of every hour in their lower gears, as the pros do, most amateurs get caught in what we call *the moderate-intensity rut*, doing almost every workout in an intensity no-man's-land between easy and hard.

It is very likely that you, too, are caught in the moderate-intensity rut. As coaches, we seldom encounter a nonelite triathlete who is already balancing his or her training intensities optimally. Even those who know they *should* do the lion's share of their training at low intensity tend to do too much at moderate intensity, for the simple reason that they don't really know the difference, a phenomenon we refer to as *intensity blindness*.

Exercise physiologists place the border between low and moderate intensity at the *ventilatory threshold (VT)*, which is the level of exertion at which the breathing rate spikes. In a typical trained triathlete, this threshold falls somewhere around 78 percent of maximum heart rate. The significance of the ventilatory threshold is that exercising even slightly above it is far more taxing to the nervous system than is exercising below it. This does not mean that exercising at moderate or high intensity is "bad"; it just means that the benefits come at a cost, so these higher levels of exertion must be incorporated judiciously into the training process.

VT intensity is just a bit lower than the intensity most triathletes naturally select for their "easy" swims, rides, and runs. But this slight discrepancy between habitual intensity and optimal intensity is critical. The next time you work out, select a pace that places you around 75 percent of your maximum heart rate—that is, just under the ventilatory threshold. In all probability, it will feel a little slow compared to the pace you normally choose for the workouts you mean to do at low intensity.

There's nothing wrong with doing a little moderate-intensity training. But when workouts that are supposed to be done at low intensity are routinely done above the VT, your body never fully recovers from them and fatigue accumulates, compromising workout performance and inhibiting fitness development. This chronic fatigue may be mild enough that you aren't even aware of it, and you may get fitter in spite of it, but you won't feel as good or get as fit as you would if you slowed down.

The good news is that any triathlete—including you—can break out of the moderate-intensity rut, begin to practice the same 80/20 intensity balance that the pros practice, and experience breakthroughs in fitness and performance as a result. We know this because we've seen it happen literally hundreds of times. Every triathlete we coach is placed on an 80/20 program, and every athlete who follows the program we provide (not all athletes are equally coachable, unfortunately) gets positive results.

Train Easier, Race Faster

A typical 80/20 success story is Billy Hafferty. Billy grew up on Cape Cod playing team sports: football, lacrosse, and rugby. As you're probably aware, all of these sports favor size more than endurance, especially in the positions Billy played. On the gridiron, for example, he was an offensive lineman. When he graduated from the Maritime Academy in 2009, he weighed 250 pounds.

A couple of years later, Billy took up running as a way to lose weight. But as the pounds came off, he discovered that he was actually pretty good at it. He climbed the ladder from 5Ks to 10Ks to half marathons to marathons and then got into triathlon, where the same ascension was repeated.

In 2011, Billy did his first Ironman, finishing eleventh out of 118 competitors in his age group. Realizing that if he made a realistic amount of improvement he might eventually qualify for the Ironman World Championship, Billy set a goal to do just that. But he fell short in each of his next four attempts. Frustrated, he then joined Team Iron Cowboy, an online endurance community featuring 80/20 plans that we created.

We placed Billy on our Level 3 (advanced) Ironman plan, which, like all of our training plans, is based on the 80/20 principle. His next big race was the 2016 edition of Ironman Cozumel. Billy arrived there feeling unstoppable—and indeed he was. He scorched the course, taking second place in his age group with a personal-best time of 9:49:30 and qualifying for the world championship.

Afterward, we asked Billy what was different about the 80/20 training plan we gave him compared to how he trained before. He told us that the workouts in our plan were more structured, and that each one—including the easy ones—had a specific purpose. "Before, my easy days were just kind of *whatever*," he explained. Interestingly, though, when we pressed Billy to tell us whether he felt he trained more or less intensely after joining Team Iron Cowboy, he had a hard time deciding. "About the same, I guess," he answered after some thought.

When we went back and analyzed Billy's training data, we got a different story. In 2014, he had done only 50 percent of his cycling at low intensity and 43 percent at moderate intensity. The following year, under the guidance of a coach, Billy did a little better, but only a little, increasing his cycling time at low intensity to 61 percent. That number leaped to 78 percent in the lead-up to his breakthrough at Cozumel, indicating flawless execution of his 80/20 training plan.

This example demonstrates not just the cost of getting caught in the moderate-intensity rut but also its insidiousness. Billy had no idea that he was doing so much of his training at moderate intensity and no clue how much it was holding him back before he came to us. In fact, even after he came to us he was not conscious of training easier than he had in the past, but he was, and it made all the difference.

The Way Forward

Now it's your turn. The purpose of this book is to give every triathlete the opportunity to benefit from 80/20 training as Billy and the other athletes we've coached have already done. In the pages ahead you will find everything you need to achieve your own breakthroughs with the 80/20 method. We'll start by identifying the common barriers that prevent triathletes from training in the most effective way and show you how to get around them. One of these barriers is the buy-in factor—many triathletes have a hard time believing that they can get faster by training slower. In Chapter 3 we will tackle this barrier, sharing the compelling science that proves the 80/20 approach works better than other ways of training.

In Chapters 4 through 7 we will explain how to apply the 80/20 system to swimming, cycling, and running and how to incorporate strength and mobility training into an 80/20 triathlon program. Next, we will show you how to put it all together and design your own custom 80/20 training plan. If you're not quite ready for this, never fear: Chapters 9 through 14 supply ready-made plans for every race distance and for triathletes of all ability and experience levels. The concluding chapter of the book offers guidelines and tips for race day.

You are about to embark on an exciting and rewarding journey. The most effective way to train for triathlon has been discovered and it's now in your hands. Learning and practicing 80/20 training will transform your triathlon experience, making your workouts more comfortable and enjoyable, enhancing your post-workout recovery, reducing your injury risk, accelerating your fitness development, and taking your performance in races to a whole new level. You may never be a professional triathlete, but there's no reason you can't train like one.

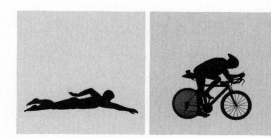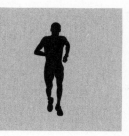

2

Going Slower to Get Faster

In 2012, Spanish exercise physiologist Iñigo Mujika conducted the most rigorous case study ever done on the training practices of a world-class triathlete. His subject was Ainhoa Murúa, a fellow Spaniard and Olympic hopeful. Over a period of fifty weeks, Mujika used heart rate and pace data to determine the relative amounts of workout time Murúa spent at different intensities. When it was all said and done, he found that she did 83 percent of her combined swim, bike, and run training below the lactate threshold (the intensity at which lactate, an intermediate product of aerobic metabolism in the muscles, begins to accumulate in the bloodstream; in practical terms, it's the highest exercise intensity that can be sustained for up to 60 minutes). The lactate threshold sits slightly above the ventilatory threshold (VT) that separates low intensity from moderate, which means that slightly less than 83 percent of Murúa's training was done below the VT, making her a poster child for adherence to the 80/20 Rule of intensity balance.

The 2012 racing season was a good one for Murúa. She succeeded in qualifying for the London Games and placed seventh in the Women's Olympic Triathlon. Having started the year ranked eleventh in the world, she finished at number eight. So, it's safe to say that 80/20 training worked out well for her.

Although Mujika's case study had only one subject, his findings have broad significance because Ainhoa Murúa's 2012 training typified that of today's elite triathletes. Indeed, most professional triathletes, Murúa included (prior to her

2017 retirement), train in groups, many of which have an international makeup. As a result, there are no secrets. Everyone at the sport's highest level is doing pretty much the same thing—80/20—and it works.

The same cannot be said of recreational triathletes, who make up well over 99 percent of the total triathlete population. Just a few months before Iñigo Mujika began his case study, Stuart Galloway and colleagues at Stirling University in Scotland published a very similar study concerning the training methods of recreational triathletes. The subjects were ten members of the Stirling Triathlon Club with an average age of forty-three. Galloway's team used heart rate and perceived effort data to determine how these athletes apportioned their training across three intensity zones (low, moderate, and high) over a period of six months as they prepared for an Ironman triathlon.

Before the study period began and at various points throughout it, the researchers put the subjects through comprehensive physiological testing to measure changes in fitness. Remarkably, the subjects showed little improvement in swimming, cycling, or running performance. Their peak power output in a cycling test increased by just 0.8 percent, for example. Galloway and his collaborators did not have to look far for an explanation. As a group, the subjects spent less than 70 percent of their total training time below the ventilatory threshold and more than 25 percent at moderate intensity. In short, they had gotten caught in the moderate-intensity rut, unwittingly sabotaging their own fitness development by training in a constant state of fatigue.

Why do most recreational triathletes get caught in the moderate-intensity rut? Answering this question represents an important first step toward breaking out of the rut and reaping the benefits of 80/20 training.

The Evolution of 80/20 Training

The reason virtually all of today's elite triathletes maintain an 80/20 intensity balance in their training is simple: competition. In a major international triathlon, the fittest athlete usually wins. Fitness comes partly from natural talent, which can't be controlled, and partly from preparation, which can be. In a race where all of the participants are equally talented, the winner is very likely to be the athlete who is best prepared, which is to say, the athlete who employed the most effective training methods.

Knowing this, elite triathletes who lose to a particular rival who prepared with different methods are prone to copy those methods in preparing for the next race. Over time, this dynamic causes an evolutionary process to unfold. In the beginning, when nobody yet knows which training techniques work best, all kinds of different methods are tried. Those that produce winning performances are emulated and begin to spread throughout the population of elite athletes, whereas those that produce losing performances are weeded out. Step by step, over the course of many years, the sport's top athletes gradually identify and adopt a set of training methods that cannot be improved upon and the evolutionary process ceases, or at least slows down considerably, with further improvements coming from ancillary innovations.

A look back at the history of triathlon provides a clear example of this evolutionary process playing out. The original triathletes were 1970s endorphin junkies who were bored with marathons and other familiar race formats and sought more extreme ways to test the limits of human endurance. This ethos of pushing the envelope not only shaped the novel events that the first triathletes came up with—such as the inaugural Ironman, held on Oahu in 1978—but also spilled over to their training. The pioneering generation of elite triathletes assumed that the best way to prepare for extremely long races was to spend extreme amounts of time training.

"There are days I'll get up and start training at seven [in the morning] and won't finish until seven or eight that night," said Scott Tinley, winner of the February 1982 and 1985 Ironmans, in a 1984 interview for *Triathlete*. And he wasn't alone. Tinley and his contemporaries were as concerned about out-training their rivals as they were with outracing them. "It seems every year the ante goes up," Tinley lamented in that same interview. "A few years ago we did 300 miles [a week] on the bike and that was plenty. Last year it was 400. Now it seems like 500 is the magic mark. . . . Each of us feels we have to do more than the next guy. I'm not so sure that's the right way to train, to improve. No one really knows."

Making matters worse was the fact that most of the top triathletes of the time trained together in San Diego, so many of their workouts became de facto races. This combination of high volume and high intensity was *not* the right way to train, and it was only a matter of time before someone with as much talent as Scott Tinley and his peers found a better way and left them behind.

The first generation of elite triathletes did at least have the advantage of coming along after training methods in the three individual sports that triathlon brought together—swimming, cycling, and running—were already highly evolved. By the 1970s, elite swimmers, cyclists, and runners had already learned the most effective ways to train for their specific events, which is to say that top performers in all three of these individual sports (athletes like four-time Boston Marathon winner Bill Rodgers, whose meticulously kept training logs from this era show perfect obedience to the 80/20 Rule long before it had a name) did about 80 percent of their training at low intensity and 20 percent at moderate to high intensity.

Most of the early triathletes hailed from a background in either swimming, cycling, or running and were familiar with the latest methods, including that of spending most of their training time at low intensity. Scott Tinley, for example, was a seasoned competitive runner when he discovered triathlon. Figuring out the most effective way to train for this new sport wasn't quite as easy as taking advantage of the evolutionary process that had already played out in its constituent disciplines, however. That's because triathlon's pioneers had more of an adventure-seeking mind-set than a competitive one, and for a while this attitude impeded the evolution of better training methods.

This state of affairs changed quickly when Mark Allen, a former college swimmer, joined Tinley's training clique in 1983. Allen soon discovered that his body couldn't tolerate the punishing combination of high volume and high intensity that the others subjected themselves to day in and day out. After a spate of injuries, he received a fortuitous telephone call from a New York–based chiropractor named Phil Maffetone, who persuaded Allen to try the mostly low-intensity training approach that he advocated. For the next fourteen years, Allen was the best triathlete on the planet, and by the time he retired in 1997, his way of training was *everyone's* way of training—that is, every *elite* triathlete's way of training.

Overcoming Barriers to 80/20 Training

The competitive stakes are lower for recreational triathletes. Unlike the pros, you won't lose your very livelihood if you train with inferior methods. Less competitive pressure is not the only reason most recreational triathletes don't follow the 80/20 Rule, however. We have identified eight other barriers that commonly keep triathletes like you stuck in the moderate-intensity rut:

1. Smaller low-intensity range
2. Lower volume
3. Lack of good coaching
4. Lack of buy-in
5. Ego
6. The natural-pace compromise
7. Intensity blindness
8. Habit inertia

Understanding these barriers will help you overcome them and begin to train like the pros. Let's take a close look at each of them.

Smaller Low-Intensity Range

As we mentioned in the preceding chapter, exercise physiologists place the dividing line between low and moderate intensity at the ventilatory threshold, which is the exercise intensity at which the breathing rate spikes. In the average trained athlete, this threshold falls around 78 percent of maximum heart rate. By definition, any exercise effort that falls below this level is low intensity.

There is a difference, however, between low intensity and *slow*. Consider an elite male triathlete who is capable of running 10 kilometers in 30 minutes on fresh legs. This athlete's ventilatory threshold running pace is likely to be close to 5:25 per mile. (Laboratory testing would be required to determine it exactly.) When this gifted athlete runs at, say, 5:30 per mile, therefore, he is at low intensity. But 5:30 per mile is not slow by anyone's definition.

Now consider a recreational triathlete who runs a 10K race in 60 minutes. This athlete's ventilatory threshold pace is likely to be close to 10:49 per mile. The problem here is that, for reasons having to do with biomechanical efficiency, virtually no adult human can run slower than around 13 minutes per mile without feeling that it would be more comfortable to walk. What this means for recreational runners with a 60-minute 10K time is that as soon as they transition from a walk to a run, they are already fairly close to the upper limit of their low-intensity range. In other words, the low-intensity range is much narrower for the slower recreational triathlete than it is for the faster professional triathlete, so it's more difficult to stay within it.

The same issue occurs in swimming and cycling. Slower swimmers tend to be less efficient than faster ones, and the less efficient athletes are in the water, the higher their intensity is at any pace. In this way, inefficient swim technique narrows the low-intensity range for slower swimmers and makes it harder for them to stay within it. Hills have a similar effect in cycling. Most triathletes have no trouble staying at low intensity on flat roads, but many struggle to do so when working against gravity's resistance.

Nevertheless, even the least fit triathletes have *some* room to work with at low intensity. Overcoming this barrier is just a matter of knowing where your individual ventilatory threshold lies and going as slowly as necessary to stay below the VT 80 percent of the time. The good news is that the fitter you get through 80/20 training, the faster you can go at low intensity.

Lower Volume

Elite triathletes train a lot: upward of three hours a day, typically. One reason is that training a lot increases fitness independent of intensity. Another reason is that obeying the 80/20 Rule *allows* elite triathletes to train a lot because low-intensity training is very gentle. But it also works the other way around: Elite triathletes do most of their training at low intensity because it allows them to train a lot.

What would happen if elite triathletes who trained, say, four hours a day attempted to do significantly more than 20 percent of their training at moderate to high intensity? They would either get injured or develop overtraining syndrome, a serious neuroendocrine disorder with symptoms ranging from sleep disruption to decreased performance that takes months to recover from. The consequences of combining high-volume training with too much work above the ventilatory threshold are so severe that elite triathletes treat it as a third rail—they just don't go there. In this sense, training a lot protects elite triathletes from getting caught in the moderate-intensity rut.

Recreational triathletes also suffer consequences when they break the 80/20 Rule, but because they don't train as much, these consequences are generally not as severe. Instead of developing a full-blown case of overtraining syndrome, they are more likely to just not improve as much as they would if they did the same amount of training with an 80/20 intensity balance. Training less allows nonelite triathletes to "get away with" training too intensely to a degree that the pros can't. But they're still not really getting away with it.

The way to overcome this barrier to effective 80/20 training is not necessarily to train three or four hours a day like the pros. Not everyone can do that. The important thing to understand is that following the 80/20 Rule will give you better results even if you train less than one hour a day on average.

Lack of Good Coaching

Some triathlon coaches work exclusively with professional triathletes. Other coaches work exclusively with recreational triathletes. And still others work with a mix of both. All triathlon coaches who work with elite triathletes subscribe to the 80/20 philosophy, whether they call it that or not. The reason is simple: If they subscribed to any other training philosophy, their athletes would get their butts kicked in races, and new clients would stop coming to them!

Unfortunately, some coaches who work only with recreational triathletes peddle training philosophies that contradict the 80/20 approach. Worse, a majority of recreational triathletes lack the knowledge and experience to recognize that these philosophies are not scientifically supported. Many of our new clients come to us after working with a coach who prescribes programs that overuse high-intensity intervals. The story is almost always the same: An initial period of improvement is quickly followed by stagnation or injury.

Crashing and burning on a high-intensity training program is the hard way to overcome the barrier of bad coaching. An easier way is to trust that the coaches who train world-class triathletes actually know what they're doing and to embrace the same 80/20 approach they use with the pros.

Lack of Buy-In

We mentioned above that past generations of endurance athletes tried all kinds of different training methods before settling on the 80/20 method as the most effective. A good example is the legendary Olympic runner Emil Zátopek, who took high-intensity interval training to an extreme in the 1940s and '50s, logging upward of 150 miles per week at race speeds. His rationale for doing so was intuitive. "Why should I practice running slow?" he once said. "I must learn to run fast by practicing to run fast."

In Zátopek's mind, training slowly so as to race fast was counterintuitive. Eventually, however, elite endurance athletes figured out that, counterintuitive or not, a mostly low-intensity approach to training is most effective. How did they know? Because it made them faster. A lot faster. Zátopek's best time for 10,000 meters was 28:54.2, a world record when he ran it. The world record for the same distance now stands at 26:17.53.

Training slowly so as to race fast remains as counterintuitive for many recreational triathletes today as it was for Zátopek seventy years ago. They feel that if a workout is comfortable, it can't possibly do them any good, so they seldom train at an intensity that is low enough to be truly comfortable. For many skeptics of the 80/20 method, overcoming the obstacle of buy-in requires solid scientific proof that it is more effective. We will share this science in the next chapter. For others, it's just a matter of sticking with the program long enough to prove itself.

This was the case with Fernanda Nunez, whom Matt coached to her first marathon when she was eighteen years old. Just two weeks into the process, Fernanda e-mailed Matt with a concern. "Sometimes it feels like I'm just doing TOO MUCH slow stuff," she wrote. "Is that normal?" Matt assured Fernanda it was normal to doubt the 80/20 method initially and counseled patience. Sixteen weeks later, Fernanda completed her marathon in 3:44, well below her goal time of four hours. In a thank-you message to Matt, she wrote, "It was the first time in my life I trained for a race without getting a serious injury and I'm just so thankful!"

Ego

Triathletes are naturally competitive, not only in races but in training too. Their ego doesn't like being in the slowest lane at Masters swim practices or being passed by strangers on bike rides or falling behind in group runs or posting really slow times on Strava. This natural pridefulness is another factor that impels recreational triathletes to push too hard on "easy" days.

Indeed, for some athletes, ego is the single biggest obstacle to 80/20 training. One such athlete is David's client John Callos from Santa Barbara. John hired David to coach him in 2008, following a series of overuse injuries. After reviewing his training records, David told John he needed to slow down. This message did not go over well initially.

"I was the type of person who, if you passed me on a bike ride, I would pass you back," he says. "I didn't care if it was [four-time Tour de France champion] Chris Froome. I couldn't handle it."

After a disastrous performance at Ultraman Canada in 2010, where John achieved the dubious distinction of posting the slowest official time in the history of the event (athletes who fail to make a time cutoff are disqualified and don't get an official time), John finally decided to check his ego and heed David's advice. At the Ultraman World Championship in Hawaii the following year, John covered the same distance nearly *five hours* faster than he had in Canada. John is living proof that even the most prideful athlete can overcome the ego barrier to effective 80/20 training by just giving it a chance.

The Natural-Pace Compromise

Every swimmer has a preferred swimming pace, every cyclist a preferred cycling pace, and every runner a preferred running pace. And every triathlete has all three. A preferred pace is simply the pace an athlete naturally adopts when completing a predetermined distance or duration without a specific goal in mind. Research has shown that most people, athletes and nonathletes alike, automatically adopt a preferred pace that places them at or slightly above the ventilatory threshold—in other words, at moderate intensity.

In a 1994 study, for example, scientists at the University of Georgia asked a group of fit young men and a group of unfit young men to ride bikes for 20 minutes at their preferred pace. Members of the unfit group spent the entire 20 minutes above the ventilatory threshold, while the fit group started slightly below it but soon drifted above it and completed the session at moderate intensity.

Interestingly, whereas the unfit men rode at a slightly higher physiological intensity than the fit men, both groups gave the same subjective ratings of perceived effort (RPE) throughout the 20-minute ride. The commonly used Borg Scale of perceived effort ranges from 6 ("This is so easy, I feel I could go all day") to 20 ("I'm working as hard as I possibly can and I need to stop immediately"). Fit and unfit subjects alike reported an average RPE of 12.5 during the self-paced bike ride.

These findings suggest it is not physiology that determines an individual's preferred pace but perceived effort. In other words, people pace themselves by *feel* in unstructured workouts of a predetermined distance or duration. And the specific effort they choose is one that feels neither easy nor hard but in between. Numerous experiments similar to the University of Georgia study just described have found that people gravitate to an RPE of around 12.5, which falls smack in the middle of the Borg Scale.

But why? Our theory is that when athletes do an unstructured workout of a predetermined distance or duration, there are two competing instincts at play. On the one hand, the athletes want to get the workout over with. This instinct pushes them to go faster. On the other hand, the athletes don't want to suffer. This instinct puts the brakes on them. When the athletes compromise between these competing instincts, they choose a moderate intensity.

Whether this theory is correct or not, it is a certainty that athletes cannot achieve the optimal 80/20 intensity balance by routinely doing their ostensibly low-intensity workouts at their preferred pace. (The only exceptions are elite athletes, who remain below the ventilatory threshold at their preferred pace, perhaps because their superior fitness level does not require them to compromise between speed and comfort. They can truly have both simultaneously.)

Overcoming this obstacle to effective 80/20 training requires that you identify your personal intensity zones and monitor them throughout every workout to ensure you spend 80 percent of your total training time at low intensity. We will show you how to do this in the coming chapters.

Intensity Blindness

The most insidious obstacle preventing recreational triathletes from balancing their training intensities optimally is what we call *intensity blindness*. Remember, any exercise effort that exceeds the ventilatory threshold is by definition moderate or high intensity. But most recreational endurance athletes, when told to do a low-intensity workout, will do the workout at their preferred pace, which, again, is slightly above the ventilatory threshold. It's not that they are being willfully disobedient; they just don't know how a true low-intensity effort is supposed to feel.

The pervasiveness of intensity blindness was demonstrated in a 1993 study by scientists at Arizona State University. Recreationally competitive female runners were asked to describe the intensity balance of their training. On average, the runners claimed to do three low-intensity runs, one moderate-intensity run, and one and a half high-intensity runs per week. But heart rate data revealed that they actually spent only 46 percent of their training time at low intensity, another 46 percent at moderate intensity, and 8 percent at high intensity.

Overcoming intensity blindness also requires that you use objective measures, such as heart rate, to monitor and control your intensity in workouts.

Habit Inertia

Not long ago, Matt received an e-mail from Julia Russell, a triathlete from Washington State whom he coaches. She informed him that her pace in running workouts had slipped lately from 8:15 per mile to 8:45 per mile and that she was concerned she might be training too much. Matt checked his records and found that Julia's best time for a 10K race was 50 minutes, which is 8:03 per mile. This meant her running pace at the ventilatory threshold was about 8:25 per mile, or 10 seconds per mile slower than the pace she'd been trying to sustain in her "easy" runs.

Matt explained to Julia that the reason she was getting slower was not that she was training too much but that she was training too hard. A 50-minute 10K runner has no business doing "easy" runs at 8:15 per mile! Overburdened by the stress of pushing too hard so often, Julia's body was failing to adapt to her training and becoming increasingly fatigued.

What was most interesting about Julia's setback was that she knew better. She had read Matt's previous book on 80/20 training and had hired Matt to create a custom 80/20 training plan for her to follow. She even used our online 80/20 Zone Calculator to determine heart rate and pace zones that were appropriate for her. Despite all of this, however, Julia reverted back to what she was used to, which was pushing the pace in every run. Happily, she heeded Matt's advice to slow down, and in her next Olympic-distance triathlon, she ran her fastest 10K run leg ever.

Bad habits are hard to break. The moderate-intensity rut is no exception. Even athletes who believe in 80/20 training, have an 80/20 training plan, and know their zones are liable to backslide if they get lazy about monitoring and controlling their intensity. Fortunately, 80/20 training itself can become habitual. This typically happens when the athlete experiences the benefits of slowing down, which we've described already but bear repeating: less fatigue both during and between workouts, greater enjoyment of training, faster recovery from workouts, fewer injuries, better performance in hard workouts, improved fitness, and better performance in races.

The Week of Slow

While the barriers standing in the way of successful 80/20 triathlon training are numerous, the fundamental key to success is basic and singular. It's a matter of accepting and becoming comfortable with going a little slower than you are naturally inclined to do in those workouts and workout segments that are intended to be done at low intensity. In other words, it's about embracing the perceptual experience of swimming, cycling, and running at an intensity that is below the ventilatory threshold. An effective means of initiating this process is something we call *the week of slow*.

As the name suggests, the week of slow is a seven-day period in which all training is done at a slow pace. Its objectives are threefold: (1) to recalibrate your perception of effort so that you know what a truly low-intensity effort really feels like; (2) to break the habit inertia surrounding the moderate-intensity rut as quickly as possible; and (3) to deliver a first taste of the benefits of 80/20 training. To make a successful transition to 80/20 training, it is not necessary to do a week of slow, but many athletes find it helpful and we strongly recommend it.

The best time to do the week of slow is during a recovery period between race-focused training cycles, when you're not worried about maximizing your fitness. Begin by doing a relatively short swim, ride, or run at an easy effort. Do not use a heart rate monitor, running watch, stopwatch, power meter, or bike computer to monitor or control your effort. That comes later, when you actually begin 80/20 training. In the week of slow, you will focus on your internal perception of effort. When you start the session, give yourself a few minutes to settle into the pace you normally choose for an easy swim, ride, or run. Once you're locked in to this pace, slow down gradually until you notice a palpable decrease in your effort level. When your perceived effort reaches a point where you feel *completely* comfortable, and the subtle sensation of straining that you've always experienced at your normal pace but were never really aware of until now has lifted, maintain this adjusted pace through the remainder of the short workout.

This will probably be more difficult than you expect. As soon as your thoughts wander away from your effort, you will return back to your natural pace. When you realize this has happened, simply repeat the process of slowing down until that subtle sense of strain lifts again, and then make another attempt to maintain the slower, 100 percent comfortable, I-could-do-this-all-day pace. When you realize a few minutes later that you have reverted to your natural pace a second time, slow down once more.

The reason this first workout in the week of slow should be relatively short (no more than 45 minutes) is that you are likely to find it as mentally exhausting as it is physically easy. It demands that you pay attention to how you're feeling in a way you're not accustomed to.

Your next workout should be exactly like the first: Start at your natural pace, slow down until you are 100 percent comfortable and free of even the subtlest strain, and slow down again as often as you unconsciously revert to your natural pace, until the session is completed. Feel free, however, to take advantage of the practice you acquired in the first slow session and go a little longer this time. Continue to progress in this manner through the remainder of the week, aiming for an equal number of sessions in all three triathlon disciplines. Table 2.1 offers suggested schedules for the week of slow.

TABLE 2.1
Guidelines for the Week of Slow

	BEGINNER	ADVANCED
Tuesday	Run 20:00	Morning: Run 30:00 Afternoon: Swim 30:00
Wednesday	Swim 25:00	Bike: 45:00
Thursday	Bike 30:00	Morning: Run 45:00 Afternoon: Swim 45:00
Friday	Run 35:00	Bike: 1:00:00
Saturday	Swim: 40:00	Morning: Run 1:00:00 Afternoon: Swim 1:00:00
Sunday	Bike 45:00	Bike 1:30:00
Monday	Rest	Rest

As you work your way through the week of slow, you will notice some changes. The frequency with which you unconsciously revert to your natural swimming, cycling, or running pace will gradually decrease. Simultaneously, the slower pace you're trying to maintain will feel less and less like swimming, cycling, or running with the emergency brake on and more and more like coasting. You will feel fresher and more energized at the end of each session and at the beginning of the next. And you may even find the whole training process more enjoyable.

Keep in mind that the week of slow is *not* 80/20 training. It is a gateway to it. In your week of slow you will do no work whatsoever at higher intensities, whereas in 80/20 training you will spend 20 percent of your total training time above the ventilatory threshold. Additionally, within the week of slow you will monitor and control your intensity by perceived effort, for the purpose of getting a feel for low intensity, whereas in 80/20 training you will use objective intensity metrics such as heart rate to ensure you do each workout and workout segment in the proper zone. But although the week of slow itself is not 80/20 training, by the time you complete it, you will be fully ready to start training like the pros.

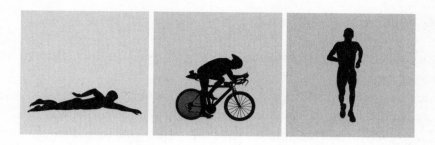

3

The Science of
80/20 Training

Although scientists did not create 80/20 training, science has proven that the intensity balance favored by today's elite endurance athletes yields superior results for athletes of all levels compared to other, more intense methodologies. Science has also helped explain *why* the 80/20 system is more effective. If you have a hard time believing that slowing down is the key to becoming a better triathlete, you will find it much easier to believe after reading this chapter.

The Recipe for Endurance Fitness

Triathlon training is like a cake. If you want to bake a cake that tastes really good, you must first select the right ingredients and then you must combine these ingredients in the right proportions. In triathlon training, the ingredients are different types of workouts that target a range of exercise intensities. To maximize the fitness you gain from your training, you need to do some workouts that target low intensity, others aimed at moderate intensity, and still others that focus on high intensity. As for proportions, the best results are achieved when low intensity accounts for 80 percent of total training time, and moderate and high intensity together account for the remaining 20 percent. This is the recipe for endurance fitness.

Stretching our metaphor a little further, suppose a child asked you to help her bake a cake and she proposed that the two of you proceed by identifying the best possible ingredient and making the cake out of that one ingredient. Unless you are an even worse cook than we are, you would probably explain to the child that what makes a cake better than any single ingredient that goes into it is how the flavors of all the ingredients combine.

Again, triathlon training is similar. In the popular media and general fitness culture, low-intensity and even moderate-intensity exercise get little respect, while high-intensity workouts are constantly hyped. Magazine and Internet articles, fitness club franchises, and television advertisements for exercise equipment suggest that high intensity is simply "better" than low and moderate intensity. Implicit in these comparisons is the idea that low-, moderate-, and high-intensity exercise all affect the body in fundamentally the same ways, but the effects at high intensity are bigger.

In reality, different intensities contribute to fitness in diverse ways, just as individual ingredients contribute distinct flavors to a cake. While there aren't many "experts" who recommend that endurance athletes include only one ingredient—namely, high intensity—in their training recipe (although there are some), the popular notion that high intensity affects the body in the same way as low and moderate intensity, only more so, does incline many triathletes to undervalue and underutilize low and moderate intensities. A glance at the science shows why all three intensity ranges are essential ingredients in the recipe for endurance fitness.

Low Intensity

In previous chapters, we emphasized that the upper limit of the low-intensity range is the ventilatory threshold (VT), which falls at or near 78 percent of maximum heart rate in the typical person who engages in regular exercise. But the low-intensity range also has a bottom end, which falls around 60 percent of maximum heart rate. Exercising at intensities somewhat below this level does offer health benefits, but it does not produce the kinds of training effects that triathletes seek. When we refer to low intensity, we're not talking about taking the dog out for a leisurely stroll in the neighborhood but about swimming, cycling, and running at efforts that fall within the range of roughly 60 to 77 percent of maximum heart rate. (In later chapters we will define intensity zones more rigorously, but these general numbers will do for now.)

So just what are the training effects associated with swimming, cycling, and running at low intensity? One is improved aerobic capacity. Measured as VO_2max, aerobic capacity is the body's ability to extract oxygen from the atmosphere, transport it to the working muscles, and use it to release energy from metabolic fuels, powering muscle contractions. Low-intensity exercise stimulates a variety of physiological adaptations that elevate aerobic capacity. These changes include a stronger heart that pumps more blood per contraction, increased blood volume, more red blood cells, greater capillary density in the muscles, heightened activity of aerobic enzymes, and accelerated production of mitochondria, the little factories within muscle cells where aerobic metabolism occurs.

High-intensity exercise stimulates the same adaptations, but not entirely in the same ways low-intensity exercise does. One example involves a molecule called interleukin-6 (IL-6), which plays an important role in supplying energy to the muscles during exercise. Studies have shown that prolonged workouts at low intensity generate far higher levels of IL-6 than do high-intensity interval workouts, and also that higher levels of IL-6 are associated with bigger improvements in VO_2max over the course of a multiweek training program. This doesn't mean low intensity is better than high intensity, but it does mean it's impossible to maximize aerobic capacity without incorporating low-intensity workouts into your training program, because it does the job in unique ways.

Another benefit of low intensity is improvement in the ability of the muscles to use fat as fuel. In essence, this gives athletes a bigger fuel tank to draw upon during races, enabling them to go faster and farther without hitting the wall. The capacity to burn fat at a high rate is especially important in longer triathlons, and low-intensity workouts do the best job of enhancing this capacity.

Fatigue resistance is further enhanced by low-intensity exercise through brain-based mechanisms. During exercise, the brain works just as hard as the muscles, because it is the brain that drives the muscles, after all. Hence, the brain gets tired just as the muscles do whenever an exercise effort continues to the point of exhaustion. But muscle fatigue and brain fatigue contribute to exhaustion in different degrees at different intensities. If you swim, bike, or run to exhaustion at a very high intensity, muscle fatigue is greater than brain fatigue. But if you exercise to exhaustion at a lower intensity, a process that takes much longer, it is the brain that is more fatigued at the end.

This is important, because improvements in fatigue resistance come from exposure to fatigue. Just as you must tire out your muscles so as to make them more resistant to tiring out in future workouts, you must fatigue your brain to enhance its fatigue resistance. By exposing the brain to higher fatigue levels, prolonged training at low intensity improves fatigue resistance in the brain more than shorter workouts at high intensity do. And while these changes may have the greatest benefits for longer races, it is likely that they have some effect on performance in endurance races of all distances.

The brain also plays a crucial role in regulating and improving technique in the water, on the bike, and on foot. Every single time you execute a running stride, a freestyle swim stroke, or a pedal rotation on your bike, your brain and muscles are communicating with your brain using feedback from your muscles to look for little shortcuts that will allow you to complete the next stride or stroke or rotation with less energy. This process happens unconsciously and automatically, and it never ceases. Intensity doesn't matter. What matters is repetition. Because it takes a lot longer to get tired at low intensity than it does at high intensity, low-intensity workouts offer far greater opportunity to practice and refine technique. Case studies involving elite endurance athletes such as marathon world record holder Paula Radcliffe indicate that while VO_2max typically peaks in the early twenties in these athletes, efficiency continues to improve for many years afterward, a trend that is associated with accumulated low-intensity training and is largely responsible for improved race performances.

Moderate Intensity

The moderate-intensity range, as it relates to endurance training, falls roughly between 78 and 92 percent of maximum heart rate in a typical fit individual. As you have learned already, most triathletes spend way too much time swimming, cycling, and running in this zone. But the solution to the problem is not to avoid moderate intensity altogether. That's because the moderate-intensity range overlaps with race intensity at most triathlon distances.

Common sense suggests that you should not go into a race without having done any training at the speeds you hope to sustain within the race, and science backs up this hunch. To a large extent, the fitness you gain from training at any single intensity—low, moderate, or high—is generalized to all intensities. You only have one heart, after all, and if you strengthen it exclusively through exercise at a single intensity, it will function better at other intensities (though not as well as it would if you balanced your intensities like the pros). But research has shown that fitness gains are also intensity-specific to some degree. Training at any single intensity tends to improve metabolic and biomechanical efficiency at that intensity more than any other. This makes moderate-intensity exercise an indispensable component of optimal triathlon training.

What's more, as we will discuss at greater length in Chapter 14, training at or near race speeds carries out a critical function with respect to triathlon pacing. You cannot know how fast you can and should swim, ride, and run in a triathlon or how to make appropriate pace adjustments over the course of a race without having practiced at and near races speeds (i.e., at moderate intensity) in workouts.

High Intensity

It is all too easy to caricature the 80/20 method as anti–high intensity, but it is not. The elite endurance athletes who discovered and model this method train at high intensity every week, and science explains why they are smart to do so. As we noted in our discussion of the benefits of low intensity, both low intensity and high intensity increase aerobic capacity, though not entirely through the same mechanisms. For this reason, it is impossible to truly maximize your aerobic capacity without including high-intensity exercise in your training.

The boundary between moderate and high intensity falls at the respiratory compensation point, a threshold that corresponds to roughly 93 percent of maximum heart rate in the typical person who exercises regularly. Swimming, cycling, and running at or above the respiratory compensation point generates large amounts of lactate, which not only serves as an energy source during exercise but also signals certain genes after exercise to increase the body's production of mitochondria, those little intracellular factories where oxygen is used to break down metabolic fuels. Through lactate and other means, high intensity boosts aerobic capacity in ways low intensity doesn't. If you want to gain the greatest amount of fitness from the time you invest in training, you would be as remiss to leave high intensity out of your training recipe as you would to neglect low or moderate intensity.

The Right Measurements

The science is clear: The optimal training recipe for endurance fitness includes work at low, moderate, and high intensities. These are the ingredients of an effective triathlon training program. Our next step is to determine the right proportions—in other words, to figure out how to balance these three intensities for best results. Science helps us here, too.

Each exercise intensity—low, moderate, and high—has what's known as a *dose response relationship* with endurance fitness. This simply means that the degree to which a given intensity affects endurance performance depends on the amount of exercise you do at that intensity. For example, you wouldn't expect 1 minute per day of moderate-intensity exercise to produce the same results as 20 minutes per day at the same intensity. The *maximally effective dose* of a certain intensity is the amount of it that fully realizes the potential benefits of training at that intensity. Think of it as the Goldilocks Zone: neither too little nor too much, but just right to actualize 100 percent of that intensity's potential to enhance endurance fitness.

Each specific intensity has its own dose-response curve, meaning the maximally effective dose of low-intensity exercise is not the same as the maximally effective doses of moderate- and high-intensity exercise. (For reasons we'll address momentarily, moderate and high intensity belong in the same bucket in this regard.) In our effort to identify the optimal balance of training intensities, therefore, it's useful to look at the maximally effective dose of each.

One thing we know for sure about high-intensity training is that a little goes a long way. This has been demonstrated most powerfully by the work of Martin Gibala, an exercise physiologist at McMaster University in Canada. In a 2014 review of his findings, Gibala wrote, "As little as [three high-intensity interval training] sessions per week, involving ≤10 min of intense exercise within a time commitment of ≤30 min per session, including warm-up, recovery between intervals and cool down, has been shown to improve aerobic capacity, skeletal muscle oxidative capacity, exercise tolerance and markers of disease risk after only a few weeks in both healthy individuals and people with cardiometabolic disorders."

The reason such small doses of high-intensity exercise can have such dramatic effects is that high-intensity exercise is very stressful. The word *stress* has negative connotations, but it's impossible to get fitter without it. The specific forms of physiological stress that exercise imposes—such as depletion of muscle fuel sources and free-radical damage to muscle fibers—trigger adaptive responses that improve fitness. High-intensity exercise doles out more stress in less time than does low-intensity exercise, and this makes it a more efficient fitness builder.

The stressfulness of high-intensity exercise is a double-edged sword, however. Whereas a little of it goes a long way, the body simply can't handle a lot of it. The physiological disruptions caused by a high-intensity workout take a long time to recover from compared to those caused by low-intensity exercise. In a 2012 study published in the journal *Hormones*, researchers at the University of North Carolina and Cal State Fullerton found that twelve hours after a high-intensity workout, thyroid function was still disrupted in highly trained male subjects, whereas twelve hours after an easy workout, thyroid function was back to normal. The thyroid gland is involved in regulating metabolism, and chronic disruption of thyroid function through exercise is known to cause athletes to stop adapting to their training and lose fitness and performance capacity, the phenomenon known as overtraining.

The implication of this study is that it takes a lot less high-intensity exercise than it does low-intensity exercise to reach the threshold of overtraining, and other research bears this out. In a 1999 study, for example, scientists at the University of Lille, France, subjected eight high-level runners to three sequential periods of training, each lasting four weeks. In the first period, the runners did six runs per week, all at low intensity. For the next four weeks, they did three low-intensity runs, one moderate-intensity run, and one high-intensity run per week. And during the final four-week period, the runners did three low-intensity runs and three high-intensity runs per week. At the end of each training period, the subjects underwent a VO_2max test to assess the effects of their recent training on their fitness.

The researchers found that, on average, the runners' VO_2max scores were highest after the second period, during which they did close to 80 percent of their training at low intensity, and were lowest after the third period, when almost 50 percent of their total training time was spent at high intensity. The authors of the study, which was published in *Medicine & Science in Sports & Exercise*, also found that circulating levels of the stress hormone norepinephrine were significantly elevated after the third training period, an indication that the training was too stressful for the runners to adapt to beneficially.

As a general principle, the higher the intensity of exercise, the more stressful it is to the body and the less of it the body can tolerate. But stress does not increase linearly with intensity. There is evidence that an abrupt jump in stressfulness occurs at the ventilatory threshold, which, you will recall, marks the boundary between low intensity and moderate intensity. This appears to happen because the brain is required to activate large numbers of fast-twitch muscle fibers when this threshold is crossed. As a result, it takes the nervous system longer to recover following workouts that include work at or above the VT.

Evidence of this comes from another study led by the 80/20 Rule's discoverer, Stephen Seiler. Nine highly trained runners and eight fit young nonathletes were required to complete a series of runs, some of them below the ventilatory threshold (low intensity), others right at the VT (moderate intensity), and one above it (high intensity). After each workout, Seiler and his colleagues measured heart rate variability (subtle variations in the heart's rhythm), which is an indicator of stress in the autonomic nervous system, a key player in postexercise recovery. They found that even after two hours of low-intensity running, autonomic stress was minimal, whereas both moderate-intensity and high-intensity running increased stress markers significantly and equally.

This is why we stated that moderate- and high-intensity exercise belong in the same bucket where dosing is concerned—they are both far more stressful than low-intensity exercise, and therefore the maximally effective dose of each is much lower than the maximally effective dose of low-intensity exercise. What all this science is telling us is that the *combined* contribution of high-intensity and moderate-intensity exercise to a program designed to maximize endurance fitness should be fairly small.

It's a different story with low-intensity training. Although a small amount of low-intensity exercise provides small benefit, its low-stress nature also allows athletes to tolerate large amounts of it, and the benefits continue to accrue as the volume of low-intensity exercise increases. Like any other type of training, low-intensity exercise does provide diminishing returns as the amount done increases, and eventually the returns cease. But the maximally effective dose of low-intensity training is far greater than the maximally effective dose of high- or even moderate-intensity training. What's more, this dose increases with experience. In other words, tolerance for low-intensity training grows over time. In more than one sense, it is a gift that keeps on giving.

The lesson for athletes like you is that the optimal training recipe for endurance fitness combines large amounts of low-intensity work with relatively small amounts of work at moderate and high intensities. But you can't make a good cake with vague measurements like "large" and "small"—you need quantitative measurements—and the same is true of endurance training. It is not possible to derive the specific intensity ratios that yield the best results from biochemistry, however. Because the optimal dose of each intensity is affected by training done at other intensities, answering the question of how best to combine these ingredients demands that we broaden our focus and look at the effects of different intensity ratios on fitness and performance in real athletes. Fortunately, this has been done.

80/20 vs. Everything Else

Three distinct types of study have been helpful in identifying the ideal balance of intensities in endurance training: historical, observational, and interventional. Historical studies look at changes in how elite endurance athletes train over time. In one such study, Stephen Seiler collaborated with Åke Fiskerstrand of the Norwegian Rowing Federation to gather data on the training methods of elite rowers between 1971 and 2000. They discovered that, over the course of this time period, the amount of training time spent at low intensity increased by 66 percent, while time spent at high intensity decreased by 60 percent (this particular study did not distinguish moderate-intensity training from high). Elite rowers in the early 1970s maintained a 50/50 balance of low and high intensity. By 2000, the balance had shifted to 75/25. (It has since shifted even further in favor of low intensity.)

This evolution would mean little if it did not correspond to improvements in fitness and performance, but it did. Over the same thirty-year time span, the VO_2max scores of elite rowers increased by 12 percent and their average power output in a six-minute rowing ergometer test increased by 10 percent. Rowing is not triathlon, of course, but endurance fitness is fundamentally the same across disciplines, and similar historical trends are known to have occurred (albeit somewhat earlier) in triathlon's constituent sports of swimming, cycling, and running.

Observational studies correlate training patterns with performance in a particular population. In 2010, Stephen Seiler led a study of this kind whose subjects were nine recreational triathletes preparing for an Ironman triathlon. Seiler and his colleagues tracked the amounts and proportions of time these athletes swam, cycled, and ran at low, moderate, and high intensity during eighteen weeks leading up to the competition. After the race, they conducted statistical analyses in search of associations between specific training patterns and performance. They found that the athletes who spent the highest percentage of their total training time at low intensity achieved the fastest Ironman finishing times. And yes, that percentage was very close to 80. Seiler's team concluded, "Performing about 75% to 80% of all training sessions at an intensity below the [ventilatory threshold] might maximize performance combined with a certain degree of moderate to intense training."

The most powerful evidence in favor of doing 80 percent of endurance training at low intensity and 20 percent at moderate and high intensities comes from interventional studies, in which the training of athletes is actively manipulated by researchers. Interventional studies involving runners, cyclists, cross-country skiers, and triathletes have shown that 80/20 training yields greater improvement in performance compared to other ways of balancing intensity.

In 2014, for example, scientists at Stirling University manipulated the training of competitive cyclists for six weeks. Half of the subjects did 80 percent of their training at low intensity and 20 percent at high intensity and the other half did 57 percent of their training at low intensity, 36 percent at moderate intensity, and 7 percent at high intensity, as is more typical of recreational endurance athletes. After six weeks, the subjects backed off their training for four weeks to reset their fitness and then switched programs. Before and after each six-week training block, all of the cyclists completed a 40 km time trial. On average, performance in this test improved by 2.3 percent after 80/20 training (a significant amount for already fit athletes) and by just 0.4 percent after typical training. The winner: 80/20.

You might be wondering why the 80/20 training protocol in this study included no work at moderate intensity (remember the "20" in 80/20 refers to moderate and high intensity combined). The reason is that some scientists—including the authors of the study just described—are interested in a particular variation of 80/20 training known as polarized training, so named because it eschews moderate intensity altogether. Up to this point we have glossed over the question of how the 20 part of 80/20 should be distributed between moderate and high intensity. Advocates of polarized training argue that it should all go to high intensity, and there is some evidence to support their perspective.

In 2014, scientists at the University of Salzburg conducted a study in which triathletes and other endurance athletes were separated into four groups and each group trained according to a different intensity breakdown for nine weeks. Two of these groups followed the 80/20 Rule, but in distinct ways. Members of a "Polarized" group were given a program intended to place them at low intensity 80 percent of the time, at moderate intensity 0 percent of the time, and at high intensity 20 percent of the time. (Because intensity zones are fluid, the athletes actually spent a small amount of time at moderate intensity). Members of a "High Volume" group, meanwhile, were given a program intended to place them at low intensity 80 percent of the time, at moderate intensity 20 percent of the time, and at high intensity 0 percent of the time. All of the athletes were subjected to fitness and performance testing before and after the nine-week intervention. On average, members of the Polarized (80/0/20) group showed significantly greater improvement in these tests than did members of the High Volume (80/20/0) group.

These results need to be interpreted with caution, however, because the specific tests chosen (a VO_2max test and an incremental exercise test to exhaustion) are themselves completed at high intensity and are rather different from real-world races and time trials. Also, *nobody* thinks it's a good idea to avoid high intensity completely as the High Volume athletes in this study were required to do. Other research with more real-world relevance suggests that polarized training confers no advantage compared to an 80/20 program in which moderate and high intensity are balanced fairly evenly.

As much as we love science, we feel it's best to follow the example of the world's best triathletes, who adhere to an 80/20 training balance without polarization, with sprint- and Olympic-distance specialists favoring high intensity a little more than moderate and with long-distance specialists tipping the balance toward moderate intensity. One thing is certain: Moderate- and high-intensity training together should account for about 20 percent of total training time for all triathletes. It is simply impossible to look at the evidence, as we have just done, and conclude otherwise.

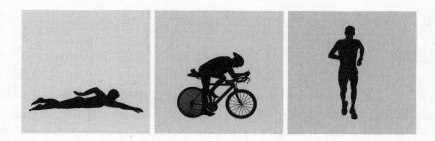

4

Swimming the 80/20 Way

Swimming is the reason there aren't more triathletes. Many people who already run and who know how to ride a bike just don't feel comfortable in the water. If you have one weakness (not donut-related), it's probably swimming. The nice thing about being a relatively weak swimmer, though, is that there is a lot of room to improve. The surest way to improve your swimming is—you guessed it—to swim the 80/20 way, doing 80 percent of your pool (and open-water) training at low intensity and the remaining 20 percent at moderate to high intensity.

The first step in this process is to define low, moderate, and high swim intensities as they relate to you. Recall that the boundary between low and moderate intensity falls at the ventilatory threshold (VT), where a spike in the breathing rate occurs. The only way to determine this threshold directly—not just for swimming but for cycling and running as well—is to exercise while breathing into a mask that collects exhaled gases in a laboratory environment. What's more, there is no practical way to monitor the breathing rate during swimming to ensure you're under or over this threshold when you're supposed to be. Fortunately, it is possible to identify the ventilatory threshold indirectly through simple field tests. Even better, these tests allow athletes to correlate the VT with metrics, such as pace and heart rate, that are easily monitored during training.

The most reliable field tests for use in identifying appropriate individual training intensities are those that pinpoint the lactate threshold (LT). Because there is a consistent relationship between the lactate and ventilatory thresholds, finding the lactate threshold through field testing allows you to easily calculate your VT as well as a full range of personal intensity zones that can be used to ensure you do every workout at the right intensity.

LACTATE THRESHOLD

You may recall that the lactate threshold is defined as the exercise intensity at which lactate, an intermediate product of glucose metabolism, begins to accumulate in the blood. In practical terms, it's the highest exercise intensity that can be sustained for up to 60 minutes.

Although monitoring the blood lactate concentration during exercise isn't much easier than monitoring the breathing rate, this isn't a problem. Lactate threshold field tests are designed to reveal your pace, power, or heart rate at LT intensity, allowing you to use these more practical intensity metrics to regulate your effort in workouts. Different ways of measuring intensity are preferable in swimming, cycling, and running. For swimming, heart rate monitoring is impractical and in-water power measurement technology is currently unavailable. This leaves pace as the preferred intensity metric for swimming. The field test we describe in the next section will identify your lactate threshold swim pace (LTSP), and the result will be used to calculate pace-based intensity zones to use in all of your swim workouts.

Lactate Threshold Swim Pace

An established method to determine LTSP is the *critical velocity* (CV) protocol. LTSP and CV are different ways of expressing the same thing: the rate at which you swim at lactate threshold intensity. LTSP expresses this in the form of pace (time over distance) and CV does so in the form of velocity or speed (distance over time). The critical velocity protocol for determining lactate threshold swim pace can be done in a pool measured in yards or meters (but we'll describe it in yards).

LTSP Test

- Warm up with 200 to 300 yards of easy freestyle swimming.

- Swim a 400-yard time trial (in other words, try to cover 400 yards in the least time possible).

- Rest for 2 minutes and then swim a 200-yard time trial.

- Record both times and calculate your CV, which, again, is also your LTSP.

Calculating your CV/LTSP

Like all velocities, your CV is expressed in distance over time, specifically in yards or meters per minute.

$$\text{Critical velocity} = 200 / (400\ \text{time} - 200\ \text{time})$$

For example, suppose you swim 400 yards in 7:15 (or 7.25 minutes) and 200 yards in 3:33 (or 3.55 minutes). Your CV would then be 200 / (7.25 − 3.55) = 54.05 yards per minute. Unless you were that kid in math class who loved story problems, you'll want to convert this result into time per 100 yards. To do this, take 100 and divide it by your CV. In this example, 100 / 54.05 = 1.85 minutes per 100 yards, or 1:51 per 100 yards.

The CV test has its drawbacks. A mathematician would quickly see that the CV formula is heavily influenced by not only the *time* of the 400 and 200 time trials, but also the *delta* between the 400 and 200 time trials. This simply means that as the time difference between the 400 and 200 increases, the CV decreases. Thus, the *slower* the 200 time is relative to the 400, the *faster* the calculated CV will be. If you find this counterintuitive, you're not the only one. But it's actually appropriate, because fitter swimmers tend to slow down less as distance increases. The problem is that, fitness level notwithstanding, poor pacing can skew the results, with less experienced swimmers tending to start the longer time trial too fast, hit the wall before they finish, and end up with a result that is not representative of their true ability.

Alternative LTSP Test

An alternative method to find your LTSP is to take the average time per 100 yards/meters from a 1,000-yard/meter time trial. This test requires less math and is more appropriate for beginner to intermediate swimmers, as fading toward the end won't impact the result nearly as much as it would in the CV test. (Again we describe the protocol using imperial measurements.)

- Warm up for 200 or 300 yards.

- Swim 1,000 yards as fast as you can, recording your time.

Take your total swim time and divide it by 10. For example, if you swam 1,000 yards in 16:42, or 16.70 minutes, your LTSP would be 16.70 / 10 = 1.67, or 1:40 per 100 yards. To derive your CV from this result, first convert the time from mm:ss format to decimal format. For example, 1:40 becomes 1.67 (40 seconds divided by 60 seconds is 0.67). Now divide this number into 100. In the present example, 100/1.67 yields a CV of 59.88 yards per minute.

Again, both tests can be done in yards or meters, and the result will represent your CV for the respective unit of measure. It's best to execute the test using the measurement in which you will perform most of your swim workouts. If you switch back and forth between pools measured in yards and meters, just add or subtract 10 percent from your CV to convert it from one unit to the other. For example, if your recorded CV is 59.88 in a 50-yard pool, and you find yourself in a 50-meter pool, subtract 10 percent from your CV, which gives you a CV in a 100-meter pool of 53.89.

It bears noting that because a meter is approximately 10 percent longer than a yard, and because the swim workouts presented in Appendix A were designed with yards in mind (though they are not explicitly given in yards and can be done in any pool), athletes who do them in metric pools will swim 10 percent farther in every workout unless they make adjustments. There's no harm in swimming farther, but if you prefer not to, there are ways to nip and tuck our workouts so you end up covering the intended distance even in metric pools. For example, reduce a 1,000-yard Foundation Swim to 900 meters or reduce a 10 × 100-yard Interval Swim to 9 × 100 meters.

80/20 Intensity Zones

Once you've identified your lactate threshold swim pace, you can then estimate your ventilatory threshold swim pace and also calculate a full range of training zones that are customized to your current fitness level. 80/20 triathlon training employs a seven-zone intensity scale. While the protocol used to determine intensity zones varies by discipline, the seven zones apply to swimming, cycling, and running.

ZONE 1

Zone 1 is a very low intensity. Staying within it requires that you consciously hold yourself back to a pace that's probably significantly slower than your natural pace. This zone is typically reserved for warm-ups and active recoveries, but it is used frequently in training. It's almost impossible to go too slow when you're aiming for Zone 1, whereas it's easy and all too common to go too fast.

ZONE 2

This intensity is the foundation of 80/20 training. Because its upper limit corresponds with the ventilatory threshold, it is of paramount importance that you stay within Zone 2 when you're supposed to. If you feel that this zone is too easy, you're doing it right. When training with the 80/20 method, you'll spend a considerable amount of time in Zone 2, so get used to it! Training in this zone confers numerous benefits, including increased fat-burning capacity and a more fatigue-resistant brain.

INTENSITY ZONES

ZONE X

Zone X is the moderate-intensity trap that most triathletes fall into, and avoiding it is one of the key objectives of 80/20 training. This intensity range is just easy enough to not feel terribly uncomfortable, but also just hard enough to fool you into thinking you're not digging a hole for yourself by spending lots of time there. This lukewarm intensity has minimal value in increasing fitness while generating fatigue that interferes with recovery and performance in subsequent workouts. Avoiding Zone X allows you to go harder on the hard days and gain more fitness thereby.

We don't mean to suggest that Zone X is inherently bad; it just has a limited and specific utility. Advanced triathletes, for example, might use Zone X sparingly in preparation for half Ironman and Ironman races, as it overlaps with race intensity for these longer distances.

ZONE 3

Zone 3 corresponds to lactate threshold intensity. Although this moderate intensity is reserved for the "20" part of 80/20 triathlon training, it is used liberally in training for all distances. Research has shown that an athlete's speed at LT intensity is one of the best predictors of race performance, regardless of distance, and studies have also demonstrated that training at or near this intensity is a powerful way to increase LT speed.

ZONE Y

While Zone Y is not as detrimental to the athlete as Zone X, this narrow intensity band simply isn't targeted by any of the tried-and-true workout formats. It's a little too fast for threshold workouts, which traditionally target Zone 3, and a little too slow for high-intensity interval workouts, which offer more fitness bang for your workout buck when done in Zones 4 and 5.

ZONE 4

This high-intensity training zone is no picnic. As demanding as it is narrow, it produces outstanding benefits. Half and full Ironman athletes will curse us when this zone appears on their training schedule but will thank us for it on race day. Zone 4 intervals excel at developing aerobic power and efficiency, both major physiological contributors to success at any race distance. Mastering this intensity takes practice and grit. Don't worry if you struggle to stay within Zone 4 the first time you try, as it is normal to drift below and above it at first. It will never feel easy to work in Zone 4, but with experience you will be consistently able to correctly execute workouts that target it.

ZONE 5

Zone 5 is all about developing efficiency and fatigue-resistance at high intensity. Although Zone 5 swimming, cycling, and running are significantly faster than race speeds in even the shortest triathlons, training in this zone will make you a better triathlete by making race speeds easier for your body to sustain (not to mention feel easier).

Training in Zone 5 is challenging in two ways. First, it's fast—and fast is hard! Second, because it's hard, Zone 5 training is always done in the form of relatively short intervals, and it's difficult to monitor intensity during such brief bursts of speed with such devices as heart rate monitors and pace monitors, whose measurements lag behind abrupt changes in speed. For this reason, Zone 5 intervals must be done by feel, or more specifically perceived effort, to some degree. Often, the only way to ensure that you've done a workout targeting this zone correctly is after the fact, for example when you complete an interval and are able to determine whether the time it took you to cover the distance falls within your Zone 5 pace range.

Because it is impractical to pay attention to objective intensity data while swimming at any intensity, this lag issue applies to cycling and running—specifically to Zone 5 cycling and running—more than it does to workouts done in the water. Regardless, learning to pace Zone 5 swim intervals correctly is a process. If you complete an interval and find that it's below your Zone 5 range, do the next one a little faster. While Zone 5 has no top end, if you swim Zone 5 intervals so fast that you can't complete the full interval set at the same speed, you've pushed too hard. You should always be able to complete all of your Zone 5 intervals at close to the highest speed you can sustain through the end of the last interval without fading, which means that the shortest intervals can and should be swum faster than longer ones.

A Note on Zones X and Y

You may wonder why a seven-zone intensity scale such as ours tops out at Zone 5. The reason is that in the original version of the scale, Zone X and Zone Y were not explicitly named. Instead these zones existed only as gaps between Zones 2 and 3 and between Zones 3 and 4, respectively. The first gap was created to ensure that low-intensity exercise efforts did not accidentally bleed into moderate intensity and the second to encourage athletes to commit to either moderate or high intensity. Nevertheless, many athletes found the gaps confusing, so we modified the 80/20 intensity scale in a manner that eliminates gaps and the confusion they cause while preserving the distinction between untargeted zones (X and Y) and targeted zones (1–5).

80/20 Swim Zones

Armed with your LTSP and the seven-zone 80/20 intensity scale, you can now create your individual swim zones, which are calculated as percentages of your current LTSP. We say "current" because as your fitness increases, your LTSP will change, necessitating the calculation of new swim zones. We recommend that you repeat the CV protocol and recalculate your zones every three to six weeks during periods of progressive training, or as often as you feel you are "outgrowing" your current zones.

To calculate your swim zones:

- Multiply your CV by the percentage ranges in Table 4.1. For example, to calculate your Zone 1, which ranges from 75 to 84 percent of LTSP, multiply your CV by 0.75 to establish the bottom of the range, and by 0.84 to establish the top of the range. In the example given in Table 4.1, these calculations yield a Zone 1 velocity range of 42.86 to 48.00 yards per minute for a CV of 57.14.

- Once you've done this with all seven zones, convert the velocity ranges back to pace by dividing 100 by the velocity range for that zone. For example, if the bottom of Zone 3 is 54.85 yards per minute, divide 100 by 54.85, which gives you a pace of 1.82 minutes per 100.

■ Finally, convert pace from decimal format to standard time (mm:ss) format by multiplying the decimal component of the number by 60. In this case, multiplying 0.82 by 60 (0.82 × 60 = 49) results in a pace of 1:49.

Too much math, you say? We agree. The online 80/20 Zone Calculator, located at http://8020endurance.com/resources/, will calculate your swims zones easily and automatically from your LTSP.

80/20 ONLINE RESOURCES

This book makes frequent references to supplemental online resources, including the automated 80/20 Zone Calculator and electronic 80/20 Workout Library. These and other helpful tools can be found at:

http://8020endurance.com/resources/

TABLE 4.1
Seven-Zone Swim Paces for a Swimmer
with a CV of 57.14 and an LTSP of 1:45 per 100

ZONE	% OF CV	SWIM CV		SWIM PACE RANGE (PER 100 YARDS)	
1	75–84%	42.86	48.00	2:20	2:05
2	84–91%	48.00	52.00	2:05	1:55
X	91–96%	52.00	54.85	1:55	1:49
3	96–100%	54.85	**57.14**	1:49	**1:45**
Y	100–102%	57.14	58.28	1:45	1:43
4	102–106%	58.28	60.57	1:43	1:39
5	>106%	60.57	+	1:39	+

80/20 Swim Workouts

The basic building blocks of any training system, including the 80/20 system, are individual workouts. What makes 80/20 training different from other approaches is not so much the workouts themselves as how they are combined.

Training the 80/20 way is *not* a matter of doing 80 percent of *every* workout at low intensity and the remaining 20 percent at moderate to high intensities. Rather, it entails mixing together some workouts that focus on low intensity (Zones 1 and 2), others that focus on moderate intensity (Zone 3 and occasionally Zone X), and still others that focus on high intensity (Zones 4 and 5) in a manner that, *in the long term*, the 80/20 Rule is respected. This is true for swimming, cycling, and running.

In later chapters, we will show you how to combine individual workouts into an effective 80/20 triathlon training plan. Appendix A presents a complete menu of the specific swim workouts that we have found to be most compatible with the 80/20 method. Our goal in this section is to describe the basic anatomy of an individual swim workout.

Each workout has three basic elements. The first two are duration/distance (how long the workout is) and intensity (how fast the workout is). The third is structure, which is how the workout is divided into segments of various lengths and intensities. The swim workout descriptions you see in Appendix A provide duration/distance, intensity, and structure information in a condensed format that requires some decoding for correct execution. Here is an example of a relatively complex swim workout, including a graphical representation of the intensity and distance:

"250 Z1, 500 Z2" is the warm-up segment. You'll execute this part by swimming for 250 yards in Zone 1 and then swimming another 500 in Zone 2.

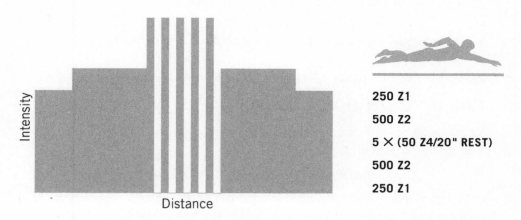

250 Z1

500 Z2

5 × (50 Z4/20" REST)

500 Z2

250 Z1

This workout has three segments: a warm-up, an interval set, and a cooldown.

If you've done some swim training in the past, you might be wondering where the technique drills are in this warm-up. The answer is that they are included in the initial Zone 1 part of the warm-up at your discretion. We recommend dividing this segment roughly equally between slow swimming and drills. Suggested drills are presented in the last section of this chapter.

"5 × (50 Z4/20" rest)" is the interval section. It means this: swim 50 yards at Zone 4 intensity, rest for 20 seconds, and repeat this sequence a total five times.

Finally, "500 Z2, 250 Z1" is your cooldown, which comprises 500 yards of swimming in Zone 2 and another 250 in Zone 1.

It's worth noting that each 80/20 intensity zone represents a range of intensity, and you have the flexibility to perform a workout segment targeting a given zone at any point within the range it encompasses. For example, if a swim segment calls for Zone 1, and your individual Zone 1 swim pace range is 2:20 to 2:05 per 100 yards, you can perform the segment anywhere within this 15-second range.

Now, you might be asking, "Isn't it best to always perform the workout segment at the very top of the zone?" Not necessarily. Continually performing workout segments at the upper end of a zone does not always lead to superior results. We recommend that you listen to your body and perform Zone 1 and Zone 2 segments at the specific intensity that feels most comfortable at the time. In the higher zones, consistency is more important than working as hard as possible within the zone. For example, it's better to perform a set of five Zone 3 intervals in the middle of the zone than to do the first four at the top of the zone and the last at the bottom due to fatigue. Only when you can execute consistently within a zone and you are well recovered should you aim for the high end of Zones 3–5 in an interval set.

See Appendix A for the complete listing of 80/20 swim workouts.

TAKE YOUR 80/20 WORKOUTS WITH YOU

All of the swim, bike, and run workouts presented in the appendices can be downloaded in Garmin .fit file format from:

http://8020endurance.com/8020-workout-library/

Once it has been downloaded, each workout can be loaded onto your compatible device and you will be prompted through each segment of the workout.

Swim Drills

Technique plays an outsized role in swim performance. Whereas triathletes can count on improved fitness alone to make them better cyclists and runners, better technique is just as important as increased fitness as a means to faster swim times. It would be unreasonably ambitious to try to compress a complete swim technique development program into this book, but we can recommend some specific drills that, if practiced often, will make you more efficient in the water while the workouts presented in Appendix A develop the fitness piece.

In 1992, Dutch researchers Huub Toussaint and Peter Beek proposed that swim velocity was determined by a combination of drag, aerobic capacity, efficiency, and power output. We won't bore you (or ourselves) by delving into Toussaint and Beck's formula, but we will tell you the practical application, which is that swim technique drills should do two things: reduce drag and increase propelling efficiency. And that is what the drills below do.

TABLE 4.2
Swim Drills to Reduce Drag and Increase Propelling Efficiency

DRILL	REDUCE DRAG	INCREASE PROPELLING EFFICIENCY
Swim with snorkel, buoy, or fins		X
Swim golf	X	X
High elbow		X
Catch-up drill	X	
Kick drills	X	X
V-line		X
"Buoy" press	X	
Fist drill		X
Kick, count, stroke drill	X	X
Finger spread		X
Swim on side	X	

Source: Table 4.2, associated descriptions, and Figures 4.1 to 4.3 adapted with permission from D. Warden, "General and specific training," in *Triathlon Science*, edited by J. Friel and J. Vance (Champaign, IL: Human Kinetics, 2013), 279.

Swim with Snorkel, Buoy, or Fins

Use a snorkel, pull buoy, or fins while swimming. These aids allow you to isolate and focus on specific phases of the pull (i.e., arm action) of your freestyle stroke without the distraction of breathing or kicking.

Swim Golf

In each lap, record the lap time in seconds and add the stroke count to it. For example, if you cover 50 yards in 56 seconds with 41 strokes, your score for the lap is 56 + 41 = 97. Try to increase the distance you cover per stroke (thereby reducing your stroke count) to achieve a lower score.

High Elbow

Swim with an exaggerated high elbow, bending your arm to 90 degrees at the beginning of the pull and keeping the elbow as close to the surface as possible while your hand and forearm sweep backward like a paddle.

Catch-Up Drill

Keep your left arm extended in front of your body until the opposite hand has entered the water (as shown in Figure 4.1) and *then* begin the pulling action while the right arm waits for the left to "catch up."

Kick Drills

Swim with a kickboard or swim on your back with your arms extended and hands together. This drill reduces drag by keeping the legs high in the water.

V-Line

Swim normally, but in the entry phase of the stroke, pierce the surface of the water with your hand slightly outside your shoulder line instead of inside or directly in front of it (Figure 4.2). This drill corrects the common mistake of crossing over the midline of the body with the pulling hand, which causes shoulder injuries.

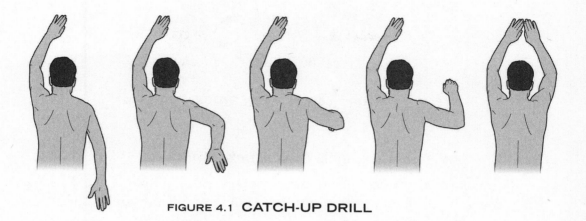

FIGURE 4.1 **CATCH-UP DRILL**

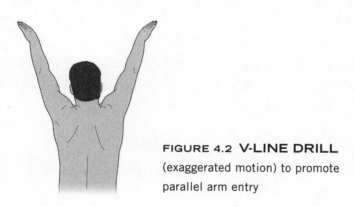

FIGURE 4.2 **V-LINE DRILL**
(exaggerated motion) to promote
parallel arm entry

Buoy Press

Consciously press your chest into the water while swimming facedown with your arms at your sides or extend one arm in front of you while keeping the other at your side. Using a snorkel will allow you to perform this drill longer.

Fist Drill

Swim with one or both hands clenched in a fist or holding a tennis ball. This drill encourages you to keep your elbow high during the pulling action and use your entire forearm to generate thrust, not just your hand.

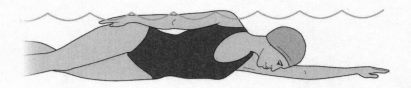

FIGURE 4.3 **SWIM ON SIDE DRILL**

Kick, Count, Stroke Drill

Swim on your right side with your right arm extended in front of you. Kick for a count of 4, 5, 6, or 7, and then take one to three full arm strokes and rotate onto your left side for a new count. This drill develops better body rotation. The best freestyle swimmers spend more time on their sides than they do belly-down, minimizing drag.

Finger Spread

Swim with your fingers slightly spread. This is another drill that encourages you to keep your elbow high during the pulling action and use your entire forearm to generate thrust, not just your hand.

Swim on Side

Swim with your navel facing the wall, with or without one arm extended (Figure 4.3). Wearing fins for this drill is best.

Masters Swimming

While the swim workouts described in this chapter and presented in Appendix A are effective, they can be challenging to perform solo day after day. Group swim classes, such as those conducted under the auspices of United States Masters Swimming (generally referred to as masters swim classes), offer a motivating alternative to churning out laps alone. But as you may well know from experience, when triathletes train in groups, most of them end up pushing harder than they should, and group swim classes are no exception. If you choose to participate in such workouts regularly, pay close attention to the relative amounts of time you spend in the various intensity zones. Adding one or two Recovery or Foundation swim workouts to your week to complement your group sessions can quickly put the ratios back in order.

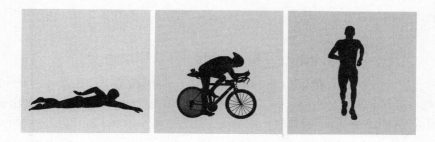

5

Cycling the 80/20 Way

Cycling is without question the most important triathlon discipline. In races of all distances, triathletes typically spend more time on the bike than they do swimming and running combined. For this reason, cycling prowess has a disproportionate impact on triathlon performance compared to either swimming or running ability. But being a strong cyclist doesn't just result in faster bike splits. It will even help you run better in races by enabling you to complete the cycling segment with more zip left in your legs.

Because cycling accounts for such a large portion of a triathlon, it should account for an equally large portion of your triathlon training. Spending hours and hours in the saddle is not sufficient to maximize cycling fitness, however. By applying the 80/20 Rule to your cycling, you will get more fitness from your time in the saddle while maintaining and even enhancing the enjoyment that most triathletes find in riding their bike.

As with swim training, the first step in the process is to use lactate threshold field testing to identify intensity zones that fit your current fitness level. The difference is that instead of using the metric of pace to monitor and control intensity on the bike, you will use either heart rate or power. Let's talk about heart rate–based testing first.

Lactate Threshold Heart Rate

Heart rate (HR) is probably the most familiar metric for measuring exercise intensity. Simple and inexpensive, heart rate monitors have been used by amateur and elite triathletes for decades to ensure their workouts are neither too hard nor too easy. Heart rate monitoring works very well on the bike—but it only works if your target zones reflect your current fitness level, and this in turn requires that you accurately determine your heart rate at lactate threshold intensity. The objective of a heart rate–based lactate threshold cycling test is fundamentally the same as that of the paced-based lactate threshold swim test we described in Chapter 4: to find the exercise intensity at which lactate accumulates in the blood. The only difference is that, instead of your lactate threshold swim pace, this test identifies your lactate threshold heart rate (LTHR).

There is more than one method of determining LTHR on the bike. The most accurate method (short of invasive lab testing) is the 30-minute time trial, which simply entails covering the greatest distance possible in 30 minutes. You'll need a heart rate monitor to perform this test, specifically one with the ability to record the average HR for a given lap.

LTHR 30-Minute Time Trial

- Choose a safe, relatively flat course with few or no stopping points or else do the test indoors on a stationary trainer.

- Begin with a warm-up of at least 10 minutes that takes you to the point of light perspiration.

- Next, increase your effort to the highest level you feel you can sustain for 30 minutes and hit the lap button on your heart rate monitor watch.

- After 10 minutes, press the lap button again. Continue time trialing for 20 minutes more. At the completion of the 30-minute time trial, hit the lap button one last time. Your 30-minute time trial is now recorded in a 10-minute lap and a 20-minute lap.

Your cycling LTHR is your average heart rate in beats per minute (BPM) for the final 20 minutes of the 30-minute test. The reason we use the last 20 minutes of the 30-minute test is that it often takes up to 10 minutes at lactate threshold effort for heart rate to "catch up" to your output, a phenomenon known as *cardiac lag*.

On your first attempt at the 30-minute time trial, you may struggle to find the right effort. If you nail it, your pace will be quite steady all the way through, and you will finish feeling that you could not go even one minute longer without slowing down. But don't expect to nail it on your first try and don't worry if you don't. The experience you gain will enable you to pace the test better the next time.

The chief drawback of the 30-minute time trial protocol is that it is very uncomfortable—essentially a half-hour race. Thankfully, there's an alternative that doesn't hurt as much. Note, however, that although this alternative protocol is easier than the full 30-minute time trial, it is often less accurate and there is a risk that your LTHR will be recorded too low or too high.

LTHR Alterative Test

- Start with a 10-minute warm-up.

- Accelerate to the highest effort level you feel you can sustain for 30 minutes.

- Instead of actually holding this intensity for 30 minutes, wait for your heart rate to plateau. The BPM reading you see after your heart rate levels off is close to your LTHR.

Considerations of LTHR Testing

Whereas a higher lactate threshold swim pace indicates greater fitness, a higher lactate threshold cycling heart rate doesn't always. Your brother-in-law with an LTHR of 180 is (thankfully) not necessarily faster than you with your LTHR of 160. Many individual factors contribute to the BPM at which lactate threshold occurs. Also, don't expect your LTHR to automatically rise higher and higher as you gain fitness. It is common for triathletes to have roughly the same LTHR at peak fitness as they did in their very first LTHR test. What *will* change as your fitness improves is how long you can sustain your LTHR. Additionally, you can expect the amount of power (watts) you put out on the bike at your lactate threshold heart rate to increase as your fitness level climbs.

Heart rate has certain limitations as a measure of exercise intensity that are important to understand before you begin to use it. Think of a moving car. At any given moment, its engine is producing a certain level of horsepower. This is the *output*. Based on the terrain and other external conditions, this output results in a certain speed. This is the *outcome*. The engine temperature and rpm gauges are *indicators* of the output or outcome, but you can't perfectly infer power output or speed from them. The engine temperature may be sky high, for example, when the car is cruising at 25 miles per hour on a hot day and comfortably cool at 50 miles per hour on a cold winter's morning.

Like the engine temperature gauge in a car, heart rate does not really measure intensity but is instead a result or indicator of how your body is managing a given intensity of exercise. And it, too, can sometimes present a false narrative of actual output. For example, the ambient temperature of your exercise environment can dramatically change your heart rate for a given output or outcome. Riding your bike at a specific effort over a particular course may result in an average heart rate of 130 BPM on a 70°F day and in a heart rate of 145 BPM on another day when the temperature is 90°F. Other factors, including hydration level, sleep, stress, time of day, diet, duration of exercise, cardiac lag, and equipment, also affect heart rate for a given output.

Given the sensitivity of heart rate to such factors, the most useful LTHR testing results are those that come from testing in circumstances that are similar to those in which most of your bike training will take place. For example, if you plan on spending most of the winter months on an indoor trainer at 70°F on a road bike with a fan aimed at you, then that is the best environment in which to perform your LTHR testing. If most of your training will be done outdoors in the afternoon at 75° to 85°F in an aggressive time-trial position, conduct your LTHR test under these conditions.

Because the relationship between heart rate and output differs between outdoor and stationary cycling, many athletes choose to conduct separate indoor and outdoor tests that yield distinct intensity zones for workouts in the two environments. Indeed, when outdoor temperatures soar, heart rate may need to be disregarded altogether in favor of an alternative intensity metric, such as power.

Functional Threshold Power

Technically defined as work over time, power is the gold-standard method of measuring cycling output. Far less sensitive than heart rate is to external conditions, such as temperature, and internal factors, such as hydration status, power is the preferred cycling intensity metric among triathletes who are committed to improvement and can afford the required equipment.

Although different from pace and heart rate, power is used in the same way: to pinpoint your individual lactate threshold and generate training zones that fit your current fitness level. You might expect the term for power output at lactate threshold intensity to be *lactate threshold power,* but in fact the more commonly employed term is *functional threshold power.* The word *functional* (FTP) reflects the fact that the method used to derive this number does not involve actual lactate measurements but rather a functional proxy for them: namely, the duration for which the typical cyclist can sustain his or her threshold power.

Monitoring power requires a device attached to your bike called a power meter. There are many power meter options, each boasting its own advantages. In the end, it doesn't really matter which device you use as long as it provides consistent feedback. Whereas all power meters offer the benefits of objectivity and accuracy, they can be cost-prohibitive for some triathletes, with many products costing in the low four figures in US dollars. If you can find a power meter that fits your budget, you'll open up some superior training opportunities to yourself.

Measured in watts, the power you generate by turning the pedals can't run all the lights in your house, but you can use power to find your cycling FTP and the associated 80/20 training zones. Our recommended FTP testing protocol is nearly identical to the LTHR test described earlier.

FTP Test

- Begin with a warm-up of at least 10 minutes.

- When you're ready, increase your effort to the highest level you feel you can sustain for 30 minutes and hit the lap button on your power meter display.

- After 30 minutes, hit the lap button again and cool down.

Your cycling FTP is the average watts for the full 30-minute test. Unlike the LTHR test, this one uses the complete 30 minutes instead of the last 20 because there is no power equivalent of cardiac lag.

As an alternative to the full 30-minute time trial, you can estimate your FTP by doing a 20-minute time trial and multiplying the average watts by 0.95. For example, if your 20-minute average power is 220 watts, your estimated 30-minute FTP will be 209 watts. This option provides nearly the same accuracy for only two thirds of the suffering. No matter which option you choose, though, you may find it difficult to execute the test perfectly (which entails maintaining a consistent effort the whole way and finishing exhausted) the first time. But it doesn't take long to master the challenge, so be patient with yourself.

Unlike LTHR, FTP does tend to increase with fitness. Every cyclist hits an upper limit in power output eventually, but 80/20 training will increase this limit, and even after you've hit it you can continue to improve as a cyclist through gains in efficiency and endurance.

80/20 Cycling Zones

Once you have established your cycling lactate threshold in terms of heart rate or power, you can then identify your specific cycling zones. These are calculated as percentages of your cycling LTHR or FTP. You'll want to retest your cycling lactate threshold every three to six weeks. We use the same seven-zone intensity scale for cycling as was defined for swimming in Chapter 4, but the specific calculations that are used to generate cycling zones are different. In fact, the calculations used to generate heart rate–based cycling zones are different from those used to generate power-based zones. The reason is that the various intensity metrics—pace, heart rate, and power—have distinct relationships with true physiological intensity. Because of this, the Zone 1 heart rate range for cycling is percentage-wise not the same relative to LTHR as the Zone 1 power range is relative to FTP. The same is true of Zone 2 and so on up the scale.

To calculate your zones with either metric, convert the percentages that define the limits of each zone into decimal form and multiply them by your LTHR or FTP. For example, to calculate your Zone 1 heart rate range, multiply your LTHR by 0.72 to determine the bottom of Zone 1 and by 0.81 to determine the

TABLE 5.1
Seven-Zone Heart Rate Training System
for a Cyclist with an LTHR of 160

ZONE	% OF LTHR	HEART RATE RANGE (BPM)	
1	72–81%	115	130
2	81–90%	130	144
X	90–95%	144	152
3	95–100%	152	**160**
Y	100–102%	160	163
4	102–105%	163	168
5	>105%	168	+

TABLE 5.2
Seven-Zone Power Training System
for a Cyclist with an FTP of 250

ZONE	% OF FTP	POWER RANGE (WATTS)	
1	50–70%	125	175
2	70–83%	175	208
X	83–91%	208	228
3	91–100%	228	**250**
Y	100–102%	250	255
4	102–110%	255	275
5	>110%	275	+

top end. Repeat this process for all seven zones using Table 5.1, which presents an example of heart rate training zones for an athlete with a cycling LTHR of 160 BPM. Table 5.2 gives the ranges for power zones and an example of an athlete with an FTP of 250 watts.

Not good with a calculator? No problem. The online 80/20 Zone Calculator at http://8020endurance.com/resources/ will calculate your cycling zones automatically from cycling LTHR and FTP.

Perceived Effort

Bicycles are expensive enough. Must you also invest in a heart rate monitor or power meter to get the most out of your bike? No. Not long before wireless heart rate monitors were introduced in the late 1970s, a Swedish physiologist named Gunnar Borg proposed a 15-point scale called the *rating of perceived effort* (RPE) that allows athletes to judge exercise intensity by feel. Using this 6–20 scale, you can quantify intensity based on your internal sense of how hard you're working relative to your personal limit without the aid of a device. RPE can be applied to swimming, cycling, and running. To use it, simply adjust your effort until the number rating and/or associated description that you apply to it lines up with the 80/20 zone you're supposed to be in. For example, if a workout calls for you to be in Zone 2, your effort should feel "light" and should fall between 10 and 12 on Borg's 6–20 scale.

TABLE 5.3

Seven-Zone Training System Matched with RPE

RATING	RPE DESCRIPTION	80/20 ZONE
6	No exertion	
7	Extremely light	
8		Zone 1
9	Very light	
10		
11	Light	Zone 2
12		
13	Somewhat hard	
14		Zone X
15	Hard	
16		Zone 3
17	Very hard	Zone Y and Zone 4
18		Zone 4
19	Extremely hard	
20	Maximum exertion	Zone 5

Using RPE to measure intensity carries risks, the most significant being intensity blindness. Many if not most triathletes, beginners especially, are not able to judge their true physiological exercise intensity accurately through perceived effort. This subjective indicator of intensity works best when calibrated against at least one field test involving an objective intensity metric. When combined with such calibration, as well as experience, self-awareness, and discipline, RPE is a viable alternative to technology for intensity measurement.

Even if you have all the latest and greatest tools, it is important that you develop a good feel for RPE, as it will help you start your workouts and workout segments (especially Zone 5 intervals, which are often too short for devices to be of much use) at the right effort level; execute workouts correctly when your devices are unavailable or not working; and most important (as we'll see in Chapter 15), perform your best in races, where perception of effort is the ultimate determinant of how fast you can go.

80/20 Cycling Workouts

Every workout you do is like a single brush stroke on a large canvas. While each individual dab or smear of paint may seem insignificant or even ugly in the moment, it's the finished painting they add up to that matters. Only after thousands of strokes have been completed can you step back and see the masterpiece you've created. It's especially important that you maintain this big-picture perspective in your bike training, which will account for about half of the finished work that you unveil on race day.

Each of our 80/20 cycling workouts has a distinct purpose and contributes to cycling fitness in its own small way. Your job is to let them fulfill their purpose by executing them correctly, which isn't difficult if you just trust the process. Like the swim workout descriptions we went over in Chapter 4, the cycling workout descriptions are rendered in a condensed format whose basic elements are duration, intensity, and structure. Let's take a second look at how to interpret these descriptions, using the example of a Cycling Cruise Interval ride. Here it is, along with a graph representing the workout's intensity and duration:

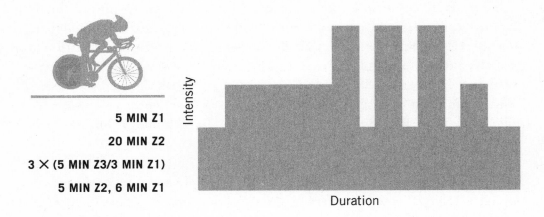

5 MIN Z1

20 MIN Z2

3 × (5 MIN Z3/3 MIN Z1)

5 MIN Z2, 6 MIN Z1

The first part, "5 min in Z1, 20 min in Z2," is your warm-up. Pedal easily for 5 minutes in Zone 1 and then for 20 minutes more in Zone 2.

"3 × (5 min in Z3/3 min in Z1)" is the interval segment. Cycle for 5 minutes in Zone 3, then back off and recover for 3 minutes in Zone 1. Repeat this sequence a total of three times.

"5 min Z2, 6 min Z1" is the cooldown. Ride for 5 minutes in Zone 2 and then finish with 6 minutes in Zone 1 (the final 6 minutes make the workout exactly 1 hour in total duration).

See Appendix B for a complete listing of 80/20 cycling workouts.

Cadence

Compared to the freestyle swim stroke that nearly all triathletes use in races, pedaling technique is very simple and relatively easy to master through normal training. For this reason, technique drills are not an important part of bike training.

One aspect of pedaling technique that is worth paying attention to, though, is *cadence*, or the speed at which you rotate the pedals. Most cyclists naturally turn the cranks at between 75 and 95 revolutions per minute (rpm), except on steep hills, where cadence naturally decreases. Beginners tend to fall between 80 and 85 rpm. This is not an optimal cadence, however. You could almost call it the "moderate-cadence rut" because pedaling feels comfortable but slightly challenging in this particular range.

Empirical research and observation confirm that the best cadence is almost exactly 90 rpm. This specific cadence has two primary advantages. First, a higher cadence delays fatigue, using muscle fibers that are designed for sustained use. Second, long-term high-cadence pedaling promotes the development of even more of these special muscle fibers, delaying fatigue even further. A tertiary benefit is that a higher cadence uses less glycogen, the precious carbohydrate required for intense muscle contractions. While sprint and Olympic-distance triathletes don't need to worry about running out of glycogen and "hitting the wall," this is a real danger for half and full Ironman athletes. A high cadence contributes to greater endurance by preserving these critical glycogen stores.

Adding regular "cadence checks" to your cycling workouts is the best way to develop and maintain optimal pedaling cadence. If you don't cycle with a device that gives you real-time or postworkout cadence data, you can self-check by simply counting how many revolutions you complete in 20 seconds and multiplying that number by 3. For example, if you complete 30 rotations in 20 seconds, this is $30 \times 3 = 90$ rpm.

Athletes who naturally ride at a very low cadence, known as mashers, often find this process very challenging psychologically. Because it is necessary to select a lower gear to maintain a desired speed at a higher cadence, you may feel initially that you can't generate any power this way, and in some cases this sense will be true. Don't panic. Be patient and persistent with your higher cadence and soon you'll be as comfortable cycling like a pro at 90 rpm as you were at 80.

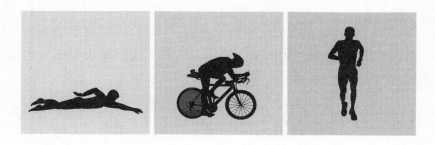

6

Running the 80/20 Way

Swimming may be the reason there aren't more triathletes, but running is the reason there aren't more runners. Let's face it—running is hard. Hour for hour, running imposes more stress on the body and carries more risk of injury than does either swimming or cycling. At the same time, successful triathlon racing always comes down to the run, figuratively and literally. Whereas every unsuccessful race is unsuccessful in its own way, successful triathlons all have a strong run performance in common.

The good news is that there is plenty of evidence that you, like all humans, were made to run, and run efficiently and long. Our species is biologically better suited to distance running than is any other mammal. Uniquely human characteristics, such as bipedalism, sweating, and lack of fur (your uncle is an exception), are strong evidence of a general human capacity for running for hours at a time.

If your current running performance makes you question your evolutionary destiny to run, odds are the problem is not *how* you run or how *much* you run. The greatest barrier to better running is incorrect distribution of intensity. Running the 80/20 way will correct this problem, and the first step, as with swimming and cycling, is to use field testing to find your lactate threshold heart rate (LTHR), which will enable you to calculate personal intensity zones that fit your current fitness level. With running, you can choose to test and train by heart rate, pace, or power. Let's start with heart rate.

Lactate Threshold Heart Rate

The protocol for finding running LTHR is identical to the one used to identify your cycling LTHR (minus the bike). It is important to note, however, that your running and cycling LTHR are usually different. It's common (though not universal) for the running LTHR to be several beats per minute higher than the cycling LTHR. For this reason, running and cycling LTHR should be determined separately, preferably at least a few days apart. You may find that, over time, your cycling LTHR increases and your running LTHR does not, so that the two eventually converge. Keep in mind, though, that an increasing LTHR is not necessarily a sign of increasing fitness. The trend you want to see is increasing output (i.e., speed, in the case of running) at LTHR.

To test your running LTHR, you'll need a device that not only monitors and records heart rate but also allows you to capture your average HR over a given lap.

LTHR Test

- Pick a flat, smooth course that you can run on without interruptions.

- Warm up for at least 10 minutes.

- Hit the lap button and speed up to the fastest pace you feel you can sustain for 30 minutes.

- Press the lap button again when you are 10 minutes into the time trial and hit it one last time 20 minutes later, when you have completed the full 30 minutes.

The average BPM for the final 20 minutes of the 30-minute time trial is your LTHR. Be sure to avoid starting out too fast, as fading over the second half of the 30 minutes makes the test less accurate. Finishing slightly stronger over the second half of the test will give you the best estimate of your true LTHR.

Be forewarned that many athletes find the 30-minute run test even more grueling than the 30-minute cycling LTHR test. If you are a brand-new triathlete, you may not be able to even complete it on your first attempt. To spare yourself this discomfort, you can instead do a running version of the cycling LTHR alternative described in Chapter 5.

LTHR Alternative Test

- Pick a flat, smooth course that you can run on without interruptions.

- Warm up for at least 10 minutes.

- Speed up to the highest speed you feel you can sustain for 30 minutes. Wait until your heart rate levels off (it will take several minutes at least) and note the number, which is close to your LTHR.

The same sensitivity to internal and external factors other than exercise intensity (weather, diet, etc.) that limits the accuracy of heart rate as a measure of intensity in cycling does the same with respect to running. For this reason, although heart rate is a very useful tool for monitoring and controlling running intensity, you may want to consider other methods, such as pace monitoring.

Threshold Pace

You may be asking why pace was not presented as an option to measure cycling intensity in Chapter 5. The answer is aerodynamic drag, or the force of air resistance pushing back against you when cycling. This force increases nonlinearly as speed increases, requiring cyclists to ratchet up their effort level by ever greater amounts to achieve incremental gains in velocity. For example, increasing your cycling output by 100 percent from 140 to 280 watts increases speed from 19 to 25 miles per hour, a mere 30 percent bump. Add even the slightest wind to the environment and the gap between output and speed widens further. Because even elite distance runners cannot sustain speeds exceeding 13 mph, aerodynamic drag does not prohibit the use of pace as a measure of running intensity, and the same is true for hydrodynamic drag and swimming.

Lactate threshold run pace (commonly abbreviated to *threshold pace*, or TP) is the running pace at which lactate accumulates in the bloodstream. To find it through field-testing, you'll perform (you guessed it!) the same 30-minute test, substituting average pace over the full time trial for average heart rate over the final 20 minutes, as there is no need to account for cardiac lag. You'll need a device that can measure pace and distance, such as a GPS-based running watch, or a well-calibrated treadmill (most treadmills aren't).

Threshold Pace Test

- On a flat course, warm up for 10 minutes and then hit the lap button.

- Run as far as you can in 30 minutes. Again, start out a bit conservatively to avoid fading near the end.

Your TP is your average pace over the entire half-hour. For example, if you covered 4.1 miles in 30 minutes, your TP is 8.2 miles per hour. Most GPS running devices will give your result in terms of pace (minutes and seconds per mile or kilometer) instead of speed (miles or kilometers per hour). In the case of the example we just gave, a GPS device would display the average pace as 7:19 per mile (or 4:33 per kilometer).

Although highly accurate, this test is no easier than the infamous 30-minute LTHR test. Once more, though, we have a less painful alternative. As with functional threshold power (FTP), you can perform a 20-minute TP test and take 95 percent of your speed in miles or kilometers per hour to estimate what the average speed over the full 30 minutes would have been.

If you already know your LTHR, you can use heart rate to find your TP with an even shorter field test.

Threshold Pace: Shorter Test

- On a flat course, warm up for 10 minutes.

- Next, play with your pace until your heart rate settles in at your previously established LTHR.

- Maintain this heart rate for 10 minutes. Your pace at this heart rate is close to your TP.

Note that the need to perform separate tests for LTHR and TP is dispensed with entirely if you have a device that captures both heart rate and pace, as this enables you to establish LTHR and TP in the same field test.

There are drawbacks to using pace to measure running intensity. Although aerodynamic drag is very small in running, it still exists, and a stiff wind can wreak havoc on your ability to rely on pace to guide your running intensity effectively. Hills and off-road running present problems also, as the relationship between pace and physiological intensity changes on sustained climbs, descents, and uneven surfaces.

Unless you train in some kind of geodesic dome, at some point you will encounter wind and hills in your run training. For this reason, we recommend that you identify *both* your running LTHR and your TP. Despite the drawbacks associated with each metric individually, when combined they become a powerful toolkit. The common phenomenon of a lower heart rate when running indoors becomes a nonissue when pace is used instead as your intensity guide on a treadmill. Likewise, the fool's errand of trying to maintain a certain pace on a long hill can be avoided with a known heart rate for a desired intensity. The two metrics are highly complementary, combining to give you a reliable intensity guide for almost every scenario.

Notice we said "almost." There are some special circumstances in which rating of perceived effort (RPE) may need to be pulled from your toolkit, such as on a tough hill that you encounter early in a run on a cold morning. In this example, both pace and heart rate are compromised, the former by the topography and the latter by the air temperature. But if you know how a Zone 2 running effort should *feel*, you can simply use RPE to find the right intensity initially and then fall back on pace or heart rate once you're past the hill and your body has warmed up. Or you can try a newer technology that skirts the disadvantages of both heart rate and pace: the running power meter.

Functional Threshold Power

For decades, measuring power outside of a controlled indoor environment was limited to cycling. Recently, though, manufacturers have introduced power meters that allow runners to apply the purest measure of physical work rate to their training. Remarkably affordable (relative to cycling power meters), running power meters offer all the advantages enjoyed by cyclists who monitor their wattage output. And because power is in fact an output rather than an indicator or an outcome, it is not affected by factors outside of actual exercise intensity, such as weather and topography, the way heart rate and pace are.

Your lactate threshold running power, also referred to as your FTP, running FTP, or rFTP, is, like cycling power, measured in watts, and there are a couple of ways to find it. One is the 30-minute protocol (with 20-minute alternative) described in reference to cycling FTP in Chapter 5. Another was devised by one of the leading manufacturers of running power meters, Stryd.

Lactate Threshold Running Power Test

This test should be performed on a running track, preferably a 400-meter track, and not on a treadmill. Since a running power meter requires a device to display the data, we'll assume you have a watch that can record average power and laps. The basic formula to find your running FTP is:

$$\begin{aligned} &(2{,}400\ \text{meter power} \times 2{,}400\ \text{meter time}) \\ &- (1{,}200\ \text{meter power} \times 1{,}200\ \text{meter time}) \\ &/ (2{,}400\ \text{meter time} - 1{,}200\ \text{meter time}) \end{aligned}$$

Let's break this down.

- Warm up for at least 10 minutes.

- Next, hit the lap button and run 1,200 meters (three laps) as fast as you can. Hit the lap button again.

- Recover with a full 30-minute easy jog.

- Wait: You're not done yet. Hit the lap button again and run 2,400 meters (six laps) at maximal effort. Hit the lap button one last time.

- Finally, cool down for 10 to 15 minutes.

Take your average power for the 2,400-meter effort and multiply by the time it took in seconds. Let's say for the sake of illustration that it was 300 watts in 700 seconds. Do the same for your 1,200-meter effort, perhaps 325 watts in 300 seconds. Take the difference of those two products and divide by the difference between the two times. The formula with the inserted variables from our example would look like this:

$$(300 \times 700) - (325 \times 300) / (700 - 300) = 281 \text{ watts}$$

Although shorter than a 30-minute time trial, this test involving two shorter time trials is perhaps even more painful, and in our view the 30-minute test yields the most accurate threshold estimates for all intensity metrics.

If you are having trouble remembering the advantages and disadvantages of using pace, heart rate, or power to measure intensity, we've got your back. Table 6.1 offers a summary of our recommendations for real-time intensity measurement in each triathlon discipline.

TABLE 6.1
**Measures of Real-Time Intensity
by Sport in Order of Recommendation**

	SWIM	BIKE	RUN
1	Pace	Power	Power
2	Power*	Heart rate	Pace
3	RPE	RPE	Heart rate
4	Heart rate		RPE

* Power monitoring during swimming is possible with some land-based training systems, such as the Vasa Ergometer.

80/20 Run Zones

Once you have established your lactate threshold for running in terms of heart rate, pace, or power, you can then determine your training zones for running. As with swimming and cycling, these seven intensity ranges are defined as percentages of your lactate threshold. Because the relationships between true physiological intensity and heart rate, pace, and power are distinct, the percentages are different for each metric. Tables 6.2, 6.3, and 6.4 give the specifics and present the run training zones for an athlete with an LTHR of 167 beats per minute (BPM), a TP of 7:25, and an rFTP of 285 watts.

Let's review examples of how to calculate zones for each intensity measure, beginning with heart rate. Suppose your running LTHR is not 167, but 162. As Table 6.2 shows, your Zone 3 for running heart rate is 95 to 100 percent of LTHR, or in this case

95 to 100 percent of 162. To calculate your Zone 3 range, first multiply 162 by 0.95 and then multiply 162 by 1.00. This results in a range of 154 to 162 BPM. Repeat this process with the help of Table 6.2 to calculate the other six zones.

Finding zones for running pace is a bit more complicated because we have to convert values from pace to speed before we can determine zones, and then convert those zones back to pace. Here's how to do it:

- First, convert the pace value to decimal form. For example, the decimal equivalent of 7:25 is 7.87 minutes per mile (52 seconds divided by 60 seconds equals 0.87).

- Next, convert this threshold *pace* (minutes per mile) into threshold *speed* (miles per hour). The way to convert pace to speed is to divide 60 by the pace. In this example, 60 divided by 7.87 minutes per mile equals 7.62 miles per hour.

- With our threshold speed of 7.62 miles per hour in hand, we can now calculate zones from Table 6.3. The Zone 3 range is 93 to 100 percent of threshold pace. With a threshold speed of 7.62 miles per hour, Zone 3 has a lower limit of 7.09 mph and an upper limit of 7.62 miles mph. Repeat this steps for all seven zones.

- These results can then be converted back to mm:ss pace format, using the same formula of 60 divided by the speed. Zone 3 becomes 60 divided by 7.09 to 60 divided by 7.62, or 8.46 to 7.87 minutes per mile, yielding a Zone 3 pace range of 8:29 to 7:52 minutes per mile.

If you are an android struggling with the complex human emotion of love, you probably use speed instead of pace when training. In this case, the process of converting from pace to speed and back to pace again is not necessary. For the rest of us who use pace, it is saner to use the online 80/20 Zone Calculator. With a simple click of your mouse, you can have your running pace and heart rate zones computed automatically at http://8020endurance.com/resources/.

Running power zones are much easier to calculate. Let's say your running FTP is 285 watts. The Zone 3 range for run power is 94 to 100 percent of rFTP, or 268 to 285 watts in this example. Use Table 6.4 to determine all seven power zones.

TABLE 6.2

Seven-Zone Heart Rate Training System for a Runner with an LTHR of 167 BPM

ZONE	% OF LTHR	HEART RATE RANGE (BPM)	
1	72–81%	120	135
2	81–90%	135	150
X	90–95%	150	159
3	95–100%	159	**167**
Y	100–102%	167	170
4	102–105%	170	175
5	>105%	175	+

TABLE 6.3

Seven-Zone Pace Training System for a Runner with a TP of 7:25

ZONE	% OF TP	PACE RANGE (MINUTE PER MILE)		SPEED RANGE (MILES PER HOUR)	
1	60–76%	12:22	09:46	4.85	6.15
2	76–87%	09:46	08:31	6.15	7.04
X	87–93%	08:31	07:58	7.04	7.52
3	93–100%	07:58	**07:25**	7.52	**8.09**
Y	100–102%	07:25	07:16	8.09	8.25
4	102–115%	07:16	06:27	8.25	9.30
5	>115%	06:27	+	9.30	+

TABLE 6.4

Seven-Zone Power Training System for a Runner with an rFTP of 285

ZONE	% OF rFTP	POWER RANGE (WATTS)	
1	50–76%	143	217
2	76–88%	217	251
X	88–94%	251	268
3	94–100%	268	**285**
Y	100–103%	285	294
4	103–120%	294	342
5	>120%	342	+

DISTANCE-BASED VS. TIME-BASED WORKOUTS

You may have noticed that the example cycling workout presented in Chapter 5 was time-based instead of distance-based (as are all of the cycling workouts in Appendix B). Our 80/20 run workouts are also time-based. There are four good reasons for this:

1 DISTANCE-BASED TRAINING FUELS THE FIRE OF THE MODERATE-INTENSITY RUT.

Let's say you have an 8-mile Zone 2 run planned, but you also have a pedicure appointment scheduled just over an hour from now. In this scenario, it's very likely that you will run faster than you should—in Zone X or maybe even Zone 3—to be able to squeeze the full distance into the time available. Doing this just once is no big deal, but if it becomes a pattern, you'll end up doing way too much running at moderate intensity. In our experience, most triathletes who do distance-based runs and bike rides routinely push too hard to get their workouts done quickly. With time-based workouts, this temptation is lessened because an hour is an hour regardless of how fast or how slowly you go.

2 TIME-BASED TRAINING PLANS ARE MORE LIKELY TO BE ADHERED TO.

Another problem with distance-based workouts is that the rest of your life isn't measured in miles; it's measured in time. For this reason, it's necessary to budget time for workouts even if they are distance-based, and this can cause you to stray from your plan. For example, you might allow three hours on a Saturday morning for a 50-mile bike ride, only to discover that unexpected conditions slow you down, with the result that you're only able to get 44 miles done in that three-hour window. Time-based workouts avoid this problem. By definition, a three-hour ride can't take you longer than expected!

3 PRECISE 80/20 RATIOS CAN ONLY BE PRECISELY PLANNED FOR IN TIME.

It's important to understand that the 80/20 Rule itself is based on time, not distance. To get the best results from your training, you need to spend 80 percent of your total training time at low intensity, not cover 80 percent of your total training distance at low intensity. Because you cover more distance in equal time at higher speeds, the two are not the same.

Imagine that you decide to do 40 miles of running next week and, with the best of intentions, you plan to do 80 percent of that distance (or 32 miles) in Zones 1 and 2. If your average pace in these two zones combined is 9.5 minutes per mile, and your average pace for the 8 miles you do in Zones 3 to 5 is 6.5 minutes per mile, you'll spend 304 minutes running at low intensity and 52 minutes running at moderate to high intensity over the course of the week. That's not 80/20 training. It's closer to 86/14 training. With distance-based training, actual weekly time at low and moderate intensities can only be determined after the fact, by reviewing the amount of time spent in each zone. If you have this information, you can then, in theory, plan future distance-based training in a way that gets you closer to 80/20 adherence, but with time-based training this process is much more straightforward.

4 TIME-BASED WORKOUTS ENSURE MAXIMALLY EFFECTIVE INTENSITY DOSES.

Time also works better than distance to ensure that athletes of different abilities get an equivalent benefit from a given workout. The effects of working out at a particular intensity are determined not by how much distance you cover at that intensity but by how much time you spend there. A run workout that consists of 6 $\times$ 3:00 in Zone 4 will benefit every athlete equally, whether it's a faster runner who covers 800 meters in each three-minute interval or a slower runner who covers only 600 meters. But a run workout that consists of 6 $\times$ 800 meters in Zone 4 will be much more challenging for the slower runner because it will require him or her to spend far more time in Zone 4. Our goal as coaches is to give every athlete the maximally effective dose of training at whichever intensity is targeted in each workout, and this can only be done with time-based workouts.

(continues)

DISTANCE-BASED VS. TIME-BASED WORKOUTS
(CONTINUED)

Given the many advantages of time-based workouts, why, then, do we prescribe swim workouts by distance? The main reason is that we assume you will perform most of your swims in a pool of 25 or 50 yards or meters, so it makes sense to create swim workouts that fit these lengths. If we prescribed time-based intervals and you did them in such an environment, more often than not you would complete each interval in the middle of the pool, away from the wall. Swimming is not exempt from the drawbacks of distance-based workouts, but they are more practical for this discipline.

One unresolved question you may have about time-based training is this: "Since my race requires that I complete a certain distance, not a certain time, don't I need to cover the approximate distance of each leg of my event at least once in training?" This question is particularly applicable to Ironman training because it is easy to meet or exceed the swim, bike, and run distances of sprint, Olympic, and even half Ironman triathlons in workouts. The short answer is no. It is not necessary to complete a full 112 miles of cycling in any single bike ride or 26.2 miles in any single run before your Ironman event. The full answer is that, when you're training for an Ironman, it would be wise to cover at least 100 miles in a bike ride and at least 20 miles in a separate run workout. These infrequent, outlier workouts can still be scheduled based on time, however, using your estimated average speed or pace to convert distance to time. For example, if your Zone 2 average cycling speed is 17 mph, you should plan a 5-hour and 45-minute ride if you want to cover 100 miles.

The 80/20 training plans presented in this book include workout duration upper limits that should meet the distance requirements of athletes of all abilities.

Running Workouts

80/20 run workouts use the same format as 80/20 swim and bike workouts. As a final example of our compressed workout description format, let's take a close look at one of the more complicated running workouts.

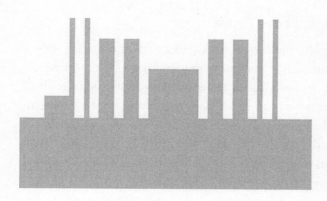

5 MIN Z1
5 MIN Z2
2 × (1 MIN Z5/2 MIN Z1)
2 × (3 MIN Z4/2 MIN Z1)
10 MIN Z3
2 MIN Z1
2 × (3 MIN Z4/2 MIN Z1)
2 × (1 MIN Z5/2 MIN Z1)
5 MIN Z1

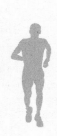

It looks quite byzantine, but it's not that hard to decode. "5 min Z1, 5 min Z2" is a typical warm-up with 5 minutes in Zone 1 immediately followed by 5 minutes in Zone 2.

"2 × (1 min Z5/2 min Z1)" is the first interval set. Run for 1 minute in Zone 5 and then recover for 2 minutes in Zone 1. Complete this set two times.

"2 × (3 min Z4/2 min Z1)" represents two sets of 3 minutes in Zone 4, each followed by 2 minutes in Zone 1.

"10 min Z3, 2 min Z1" is a single, 10-minute Zone 3 effort followed by 2 minutes of Zone 1 recovery.

"2 × (3 min Z4/2 min Z1)" is a repetition of the previous segment comprising two sets of 3 minutes in Zone 4, each followed by 2 minutes in Zone 1.

"2 × (1 min Z5/2 min Z1)" is the final interval set, and it consists of 1 minute in Zone 5 followed by 2 minutes of Zone 1 recovery, repeated twice.

"5 min Z1" is the cooldown.

See Appendix C for a complete listing of 80/20 running workouts.

Running Drills

Becoming a more efficient runner is a big part of becoming a more proficient runner. For the most part, this happens automatically. Your stride will evolve in energy-saving ways that you aren't even aware of as you work on building your running fitness. But the following running drills can help the process along. We recommend that you find time to do them once a week.

Cadence Count

The most common running technique flaw is overstriding, or touching the foot to the ground out in front of the body, which creates a braking effect. Your stride will naturally shorten as you gain running experience. Although it's difficult to measure stride length on the run, you can get at it in a different way by measuring your cadence. As your stride shortens, you will take more steps per minute at any given pace. Periodically audit your stride rate by counting how many steps you take with your right foot in one minute at a particular pace. (Some running devices measure cadence throughout every run.) Get a sense for what a shorter stride feels like by slightly increasing your step count in the next minute.

Hands on Head

You can't run forward without also bouncing up and down, but too much vertical oscillation is a big energy waster. By running with your hands on your head, you will become more aware of your bouncing and can tweak your run form to reduce it if necessary.

High Knees

The high knees drill gives you practice touching your feet to the ground directly underneath your hips, as should happen when you run. To do it, run in place at a high tempo for 20 seconds, lifting your knees as high as you can with each step.

Skipping

Who cares what your neighbors think? Skipping is a great way to feel an exaggerated and powerful toe-off, which is the point of your stride where your trailing leg pushes off the ground. Although skipping results in ridiculous amounts of vertical oscillation, the point is to feel what a powerful toe-off is like and replicate that feeling in regular running. To do it, simply skip forward at a moderately fast pace for 20 seconds at a time, leaping as high as you can with each skip. If you don't know how to skip, ask an eight-year-old.

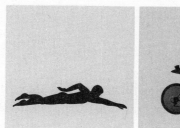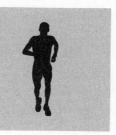

7

Strength, Flexibility, and Mobility Training

As an endurance sport, triathlon requires a type of fitness whose main ingredients are stamina and speed. But these are not the only attributes you need to perform optimally. Strength, flexibility, and mobility are important also. Because if this, we recommend that all triathletes train these qualities in addition to hitting the pool, riding their bike, and running.

Strength training (weightlifting and other forms of moving against resistance) increases the force-producing capacity of the muscles and is proven to improve running efficiency and reduce the risk of some of the overuse injuries that are common in triathletes. Mobility is the ability of the shoulders, hips, and other major joints to move efficiently through a full range of motion. Mobility exercises help increase this capacity, resulting in more efficient swimming, cycling, and running. Flexibility refers to a joint's passive range of motion (ROM). Although to be a successful triathlete you do not need any more than a normal range of motion in the major joints, many triathletes have impaired ROM in certain joints because of muscle tightness caused mainly by spending too much time in a seated position when not training, an issue that is exacerbated by the body positions held during training, particularly on the bike. Flexibility training, which entails static stretches, such as the familiar toe touch, restores full ROM and reduces the risk of the various overuse injuries that tight muscles (and tendons) contribute to.

So, as you can see, strength, mobility, and flexibility training are well worth your time. But there's the rub. Many triathletes find it hard enough to fit all of the swimming, cycling, and running they wish to do into their schedule and feel there just aren't enough hours in the day to add anything else, benefits notwithstanding.

We get it, which is why we offer a flexible and pragmatic approach to strength, flexibility, and mobility training (or "ancillary training," as we refer to these activities collectively) that won't require you to quit your job or neglect your family. To begin with, these types of training are not included in the training plans presented in Chapters 10 through 14. This gives you the option to skip them if you lack the time or inclination. There are successful triathletes who never hit the gym or touch their toes. Although we don't recommend that you follow their example, we understand it's a necessity for some triathletes.

Professional triathletes devote significant amounts of time to ancillary training, and they tend to follow sophisticated programs individualized to their specific needs. But as a recreational triathlete, you can get the lion's share of the benefits that ancillary training offers through a pragmatic approach that is simple and time-efficient.

In this chapter we describe an at-home strength workout that you can easily do while watching the evening news or overseeing your child's homework, a gym-based strength workout that you can bang out in as little as 20 minutes (perhaps at the same facility where you swim), a mobility routine that can be combined with either of the strength workouts for maximum time efficiency, and a list of flexibility exercises that we encourage you to use on an à la carte basis, practicing only those you really need.

At-Home Strength Workout

■ Equipment needed:
stability ball, exercise bench, medicine ball or dumbbells

■ Recommended frequency:
2 times per week

This ten-movement, full-body functional strength workout can be done in the comfort of your own home with minimal equipment. All you need is a stability ball and an exercise bench or something that can serve the same function. We recommend that you do the workout two times per week. If you have not done any strength training recently, you should begin with one set of each exercise. After three weeks, add a second set if you have time and want a slightly greater training effect. In this case, do the workout as a circuit, completing each exercise once before going back and repeating all of them. After two more weeks, add a third circuit, but again only if you have both the time and the desire. The movements are arranged in such a way that you are never challenging the same muscles consecutively (the words beneath the exercise name specify the muscles involved), so you can move from one to the next with minimal rest, further enhancing the workout's time efficiency.

If some of these exercises look kind of strange to you, you're probably not alone. Strength-training methods have evolved significantly over the past decade or two. Professional triathletes today base their strength workouts on functional movements that bear little resemblance to the bodybuilding exercises that used to be one-size-fits-all across all sports. But these improved methods have achieved little penetration in the age-group triathlon ranks. In the same way that most recreational triathletes do more than 30 percent of their swimming, cycling, and running at moderate intensity whereas the pros do less than 20 percent, most age-groupers are still doing such exercises as dumbbell shoulder presses (which do little or nothing to aid triathlon performance) in the gym, while the elites are doing exercises like those you see in this chapter.

Amateur racers who do make the switch to current best practices in strength training for triathlon never regret it. One example is Bob Kusenberger, a San Antonio–based entrepreneur and triathlete coached by Matt. Asked recently how pro-style strength training has helped him, Bob identified no fewer than four benefits. "It has concentrated a lot more on my core," he said, "focused on my hips and glutes (which get neglected by most traditional bodybuilding exercises other than squats), made my ankles and knees more stable, and improved my strength without bulking me up."

Sound good? Then do this workout!

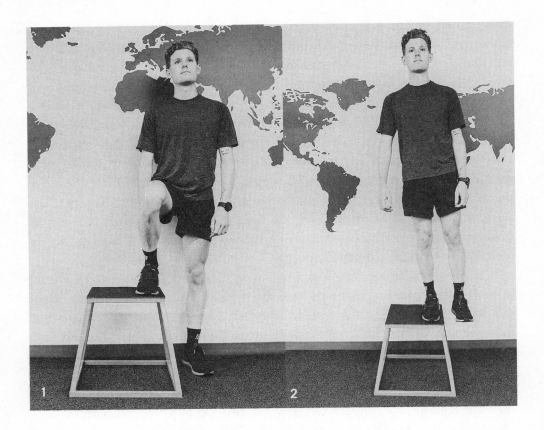

Side Step-Up

Glutes, hamstrings, quadriceps

1 Stand with your right foot resting flat on a 15- to 18-inch platform (such as an exercise bench) and your left foot on the floor, so that your right knee is bent about 60 degrees and your left leg is straight.

2 Shift your weight onto the heel of your right foot and straighten your right leg, raising your whole body upward. Pause briefly with your left foot suspended next to your right foot and then bend your right leg again, lowering your left foot back to the floor. Complete 10 repetitions, then switch legs. If you find this exercise easy, do it while holding a dumbbell in the hand on your nonworking side, completing 10 reps with a weight you could lift 12 times with perfect form.

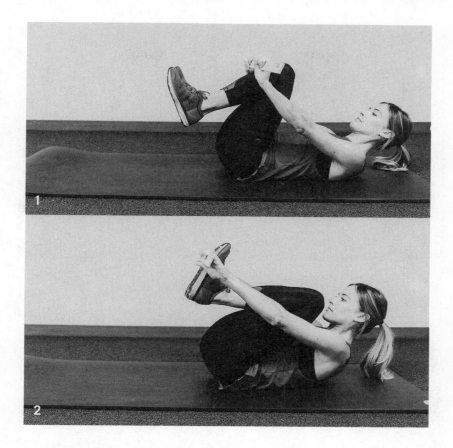

Stick Crunch

Front abdominals

1 Lie face up on the floor and draw your knees to your chest. Hold a short stick, rope, or rolled-up towel between your hands at shoulder width with your arms extended straight toward your toes.

2 Try to reach the stick past your feet by pressing your chest toward your knees and pulling your knees toward your chest (i.e., curling into a ball). Pause briefly with the stick on the far side of your feet and then relax. Complete 12 repetitions or two fewer than your maximum (whichever comes first).

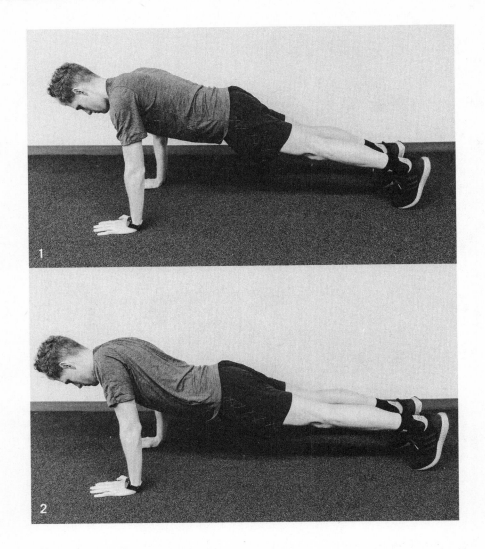

Scapular Push-Up

Chest, rear shoulders, triceps

1 Assume a standard push-up position.

2 Keeping your elbows locked, retract your shoulder blades so that your torso sinks a couple of inches toward the floor.

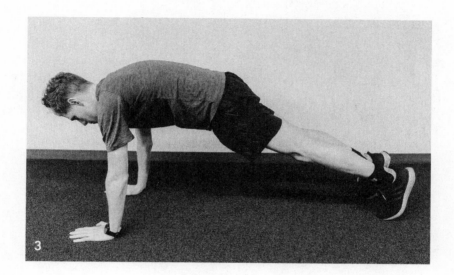

3 Now protract your shoulder blades fully, so that your upper back takes on a slightly hunched look. Finally, return to the start position. Complete 12 repetitions or two fewer than your maximum (whichever comes first).

For a greater challenge, complete a full, normal push-up after each scapular retraction/protraction.

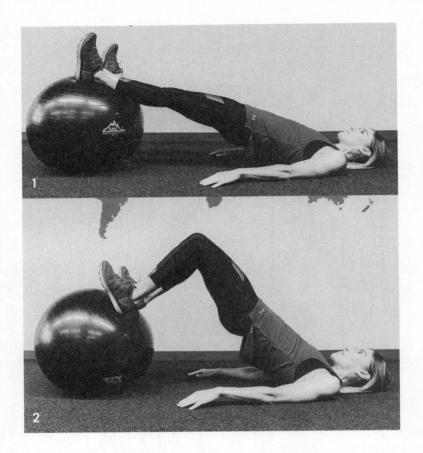

Stability Ball Hamstring Curl
Hamstrings

1 Start in a bridge position, face up, with your head and shoulders on the floor and your heels resting on top of a stability ball, your body suspended in a straight line between these points.

2 Contract your hamstrings and roll the ball toward your rear end. Pause briefly and extend your legs, rolling the ball back to the starting point. Don't let your hips drop. Complete 12 repetitions or two fewer than your maximum (whichever comes first).

   If this exercise is too easy for you, do the advanced version, which involves working each leg individually.

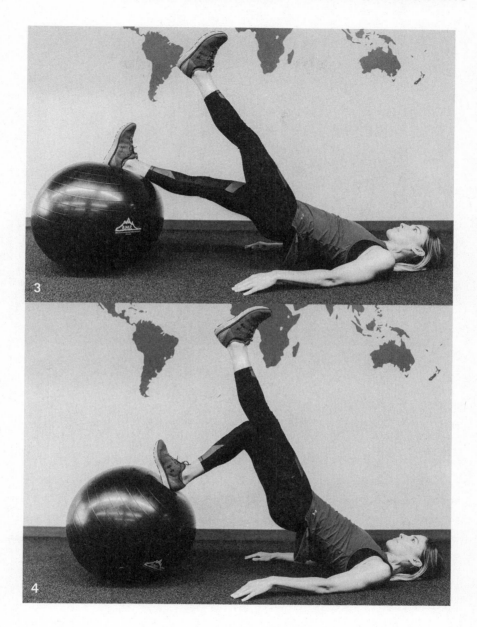

3–4 Start in the same position but lift your left leg several inches above the ball and hold it there while you roll the ball back and forth 12 times (or two fewer than your maximum) with your right leg. Then repeat the exercise with your left leg.

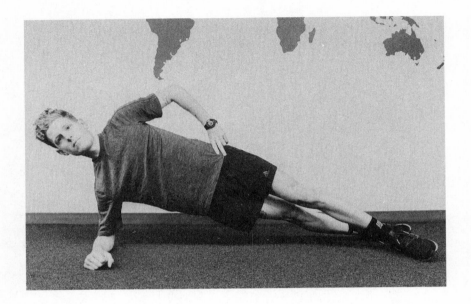

Side Plank

Side abdominals

Lie on your right side with your left foot just in front of the right on the floor and your torso propped up by your upper arm. Lift your hips until your body forms a diagonal plank from ankles to neck. Hold this position for 60 seconds or 10 seconds short of your limit (whichever comes first), making sure you don't allow your hips to sag toward the floor. (Watch yourself in a mirror to make sure you're not sagging.) Switch to the left side and repeat the exercise.

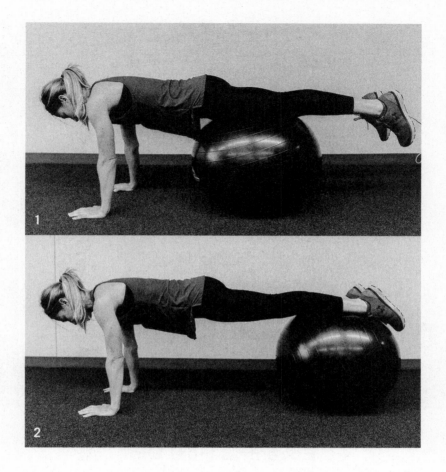

Stability Ball Walkout

Upper back, rear shoulders, front abdominals

1 Start in a modified push-up position with your palms flat on the floor and your upper thighs supported by a stability ball.

2 Start walking forward with your hands and continue until the ball us under the top of your feet. Don't arch your back or let your hips sag. Now walk the other way until the ball is again underneath your upper thighs. Complete 12 repetitions or two fewer than your maximum (whichever comes first).

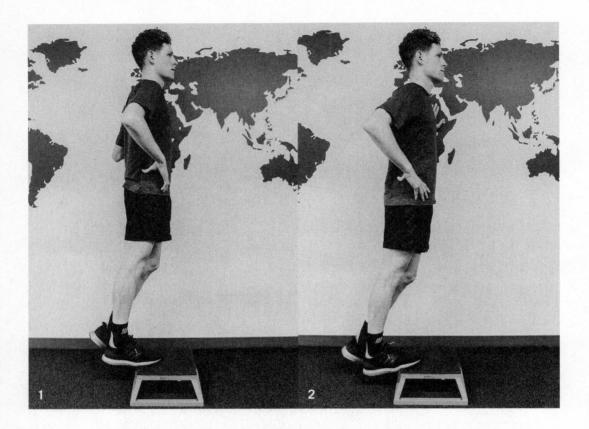

Eccentric Heel Dip
Calves

1 Balance on your right foot on a sturdy platform with the ball of the foot resting on the edge of the platform so that the heel is unsupported. Rest your fingertips against a wall or some other support for balance.

2 Lower your heel toward the floor until you feel a stretch in your calf muscles, then raise your heel back to a neutral position. Do 12 repetitions or two fewer than your maximum (whichever comes first) and then repeat the exercise on your left foot.

If this exercise is too difficult, try standing on the balls of both feet and dipping your left and right heels together, completing 12 repetitions or two fewer than your maximum.

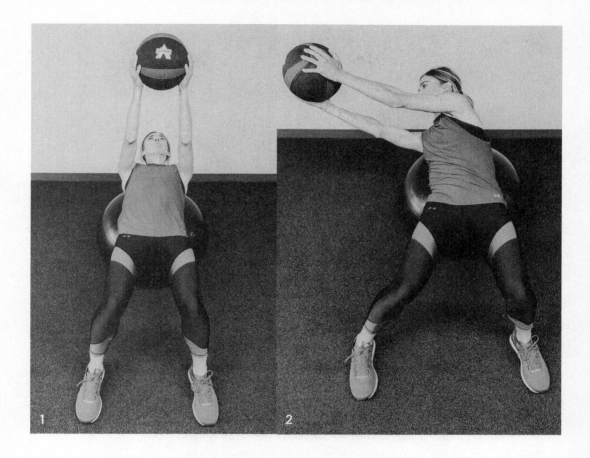

Stability Ball Trunk Rotation

Abdominals, lower back

1 Lie face up on a stability ball with your feet spread wide on the floor, your upper back supported, and your arms extended straight overhead with a medicine ball, dumbbell, or other weight pressed between your palms.

2 Keeping your arms extended, rotate your upper torso to the right and swing the ball toward the wall on that side of the room. Go as far as you can without discomfort and then return to the start position. Now rotate to the opposite side. Complete 10 repetitions (i.e., 10 rotations each way) with a weight that you could do 12 perfect reps with.

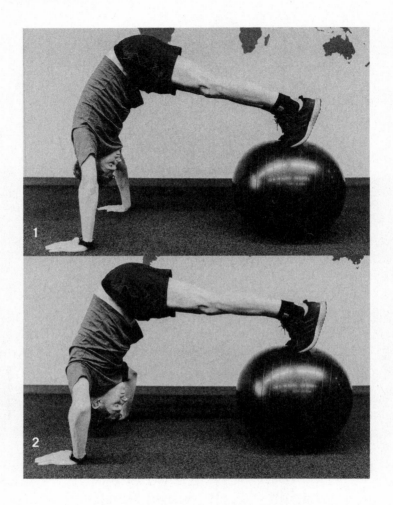

Inverted Shoulder Press
Shoulders, chest, triceps

1 Start from a pike position with your feet on a stability ball, your palms on the floor, and your rear end elevated so your body is in the shape of an inverted V.

2 Now bend your elbows and lower the crown of your head toward the floor between your hands. Go as far as you can without strain; it's okay if it isn't very far. Now press back to the start position. Complete 10 repetitions.

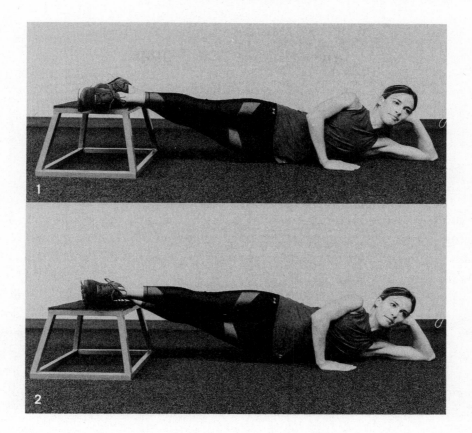

Side Lying Hip Lift

Hips, side abdominals

1 Lie on the floor on your left side with your feet on top of an exercise bench, your right foot just in front of your left.

2 Contract the muscles on the outside of your left hip and lift your hips off the floor until your body forms a straight line. Pause briefly and then return to the start position. Complete 10 repetitions or two fewer than your maximum (whichever comes first) and then flip over and repeat the exercise on the other side.

If this exercise is too easy for you, do a one-leg version with only the foot of the top leg resting on the bench and the other leg bent so it doesn't assist in the lifting action.

Gym-Based Strength Workout

■ **Equipment needed:**
Dumbbells, cable pulley station, stability ball,
kettlebell, chin-up bar, resistance band, BOSU ball or balance disk

■ **Recommended frequency:**
2 times per week

If you have access to a fully equipped fitness center, you may prefer to do this strength workout instead of the home-based workout. Similar in overall structure, it is made up of more equipment-intensive exercises that are by and large slightly more beneficial.

All of the guidelines that apply to the home-based strength workout apply to this one as well. Complete the session two times per week. If you have not done any strength training recently, begin with one set of each exercise. After two weeks, add a second set if you have time and want a slightly greater training effect. In this case, do the workout as a circuit, completing each exercise once before going back and repeating all of them. After two more weeks, add a third circuit, but again only if you have both the time and the desire.

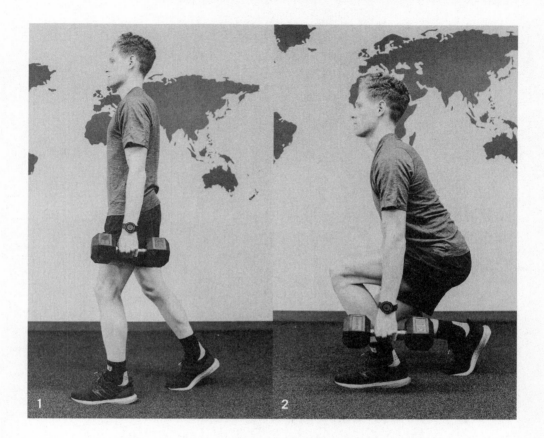

Split-Stance Dumbbell Deadlift

Glutes, hips, quadriceps, hamstrings

1 Stand with your right foot half a step behind your left foot and your left foot flat on the floor beneath your hip and only the toes of your right foot touching the floor. Begin with a dumbbell in each hand and your arms relaxed at your sides.

2 Now bend at the hips and knees (not the waist) and reach toward the floor with the dumbbells, stopping when the weights are a few inches from the ground. Pause briefly and then press your right heel into the floor and return to a standing position. Concentrate on contracting your right glutes and keeping your torso as erect as possible when executing this motion. Complete 10 repetitions with a weight you could lift 12 times with perfect form and then reverse your stance and repeat the exercise.

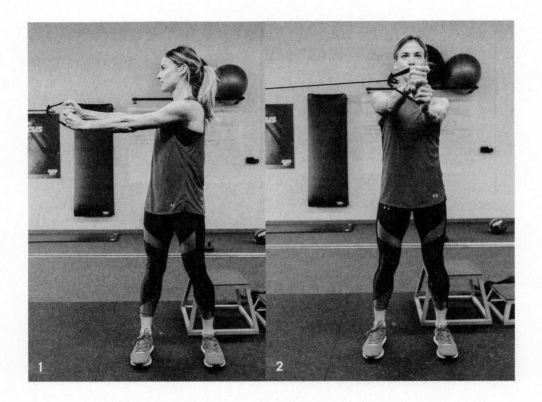

Standing Cable Trunk Rotation
Abdominals

1 Stand with your left side facing a cable pulley station with a handle attached at shoulder height. Grasp the handle with both hands and both arms fully extended. Begin with your torso rotated toward the handle and tension in the cable (i.e., the weight stack is slightly elevated from the resting position).

2 Rotate your torso to the right while keeping your arms fully extended and the handle in line with the center of your chest. Keep your eyes focused on the handle as you rotate and your hips pressed forward. Return to the start position without allowing the weight stack to come to rest. Complete 10 repetitions with a weight you could lift 12 times with perfect form, then reverse your position and repeat the exercise.

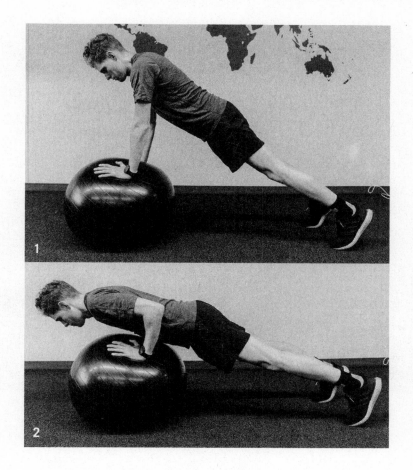

Stability Ball Push-Up

Chest, rear shoulders, triceps

1 Assume a modified push-up position with your feet together, your body forming a perfectly straight line, and your palms positioned slightly more than shoulder width apart on a stability ball.

2 Bend your elbows and smoothly lower your chest to within an inch of the ball. Immediately press back upward to the start position. Complete 12 repetitions or two fewer than your maximum (whichever comes first). If you have difficulty doing a full push-up, do a half push-up, bending your elbows only to 90 degrees before pressing upward.

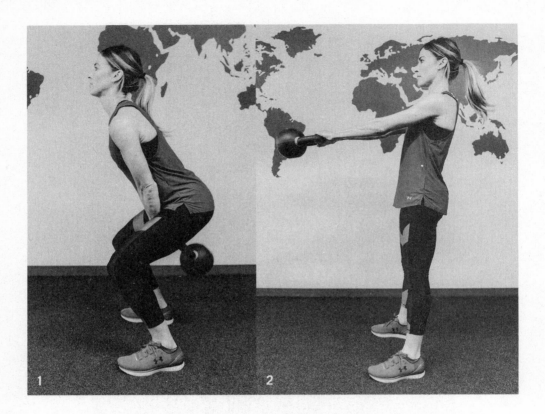

Kettlebell Swing

Hamstrings, glutes, lower back, shoulders

1 Stand in a broad stance with your toes pointed outward slightly, your knees bent about 30 degrees, and your trunk bent forward at a similar angle from the hips, not the waist. Begin with both hands on the handle of a kettlebell in an overhand grip, elbows straight and the weight hanging between your knees.

2 Keeping your spine neutral, snap your hips forward and use the momentum generated by this action to swing the kettlebell out in front of you. Do not use your back or shoulder muscles to extend the arc of this swing. If the weight comes all the way up to shoulder level, you're doing it wrong. Now reverse this movement, bending your knees and hips and allowing the kettlebell to swing between your legs. Bring the movement of the ball to a full stop so that momentum does not assist the next swing. Complete 12 repetitions using a weight you could lift 15 times with perfect form.

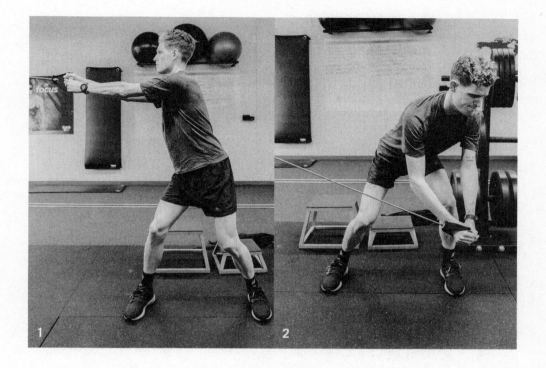

Standing Cable High-Low Pull
Abdominals, shoulders, upper back

1 Stand with your left side facing a cable pulley station with a D-handle attached at shoulder height. Bend your knees slightly and place your feet a little more than shoulder width apart. Grasp the handle in both hands. Your arms should be almost fully extended with your trunk rotated to the left.

2 Now pull the handle from this position across your body and toward the floor, stopping when your hands are outside your right knee. This is a compound movement that involves twisting your torso to the right, shifting your weight from your left foot to your right foot, bending toward the floor, and using your shoulders to pull the handle across your body. Concentrate on initiating the movement with your trunk muscles. At the bottom of the movement, pause briefly, then smoothly return to the start position. Complete 10 repetitions with a weight you could lift 12 times with perfect form, then reverse your position and repeat. It's a good idea to practice this exercise with minimal weight before you do it for real.

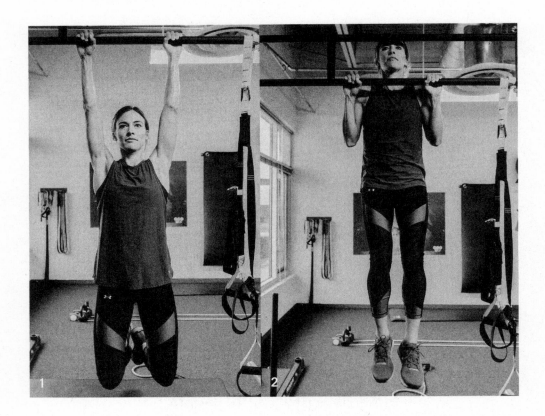

Pull-Up

Upper back, biceps

1 Grab a pull-up bar with an overhand grip and your hands positioned slightly more than shoulder width apart. Begin from a full hang. (If the bar is low, bend your knees, tucking your lower legs behind you.)

2 Pull your body upward until your chin clears the bar, then lower yourself back to a full hang. Complete 10 repetitions or two fewer than your maximum (whichever comes first). If you cannot complete at least eight pull-ups on your own, have a partner assist you by pushing you upward from a standing position on the floor as necessary.

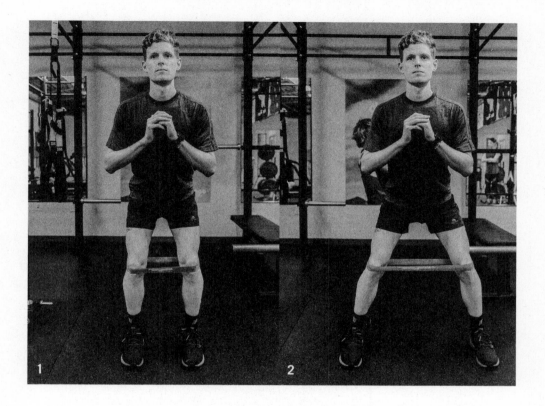

Band Walk

Hips, groin

1 Loop a high-tension resistance band around your thighs just above the knees and stand with a slight bend in your knees.

2 Take a moderately large step to the right with your right foot. Now take an equal-size step to the right with your left foot, resisting the band's tendency to make the movement quick and jerky. Make sure that you keep the hips and shoulders level, and don't deviate forward or backward as you go to the side. When this exercise is performed correctly, you'll feel the movement in your inner and outer thighs. Complete 10 steps to the right and then 10 more in the opposite direction.

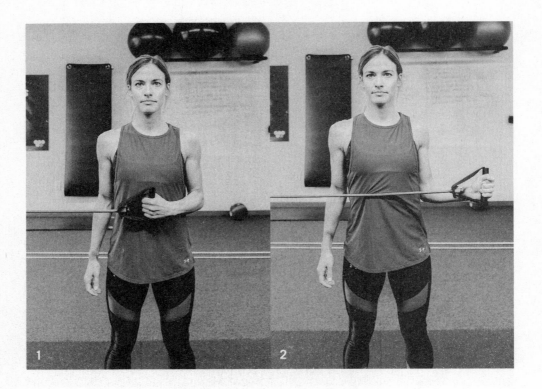

Standing Cable
External/Internal Shoulder Rotation
Shoulder rotator cuff

1 Stand with your left side facing a cable pulley station. Grasp the D-handle in your right hand and begin with your right arm pressed against your side and bent 90 degrees so that your forearm is pointing toward the cable pulley station across your belly.

2 Now rotate your shoulder externally and pull the handle across your body, keeping your elbow and upper arm pressed against your right side. When you reach the limit of your range of motion, pause briefly and return to the start position. Complete 10 repetitions with a weight you could lift 12 times with perfect form and then repeat the exercise with your left arm.

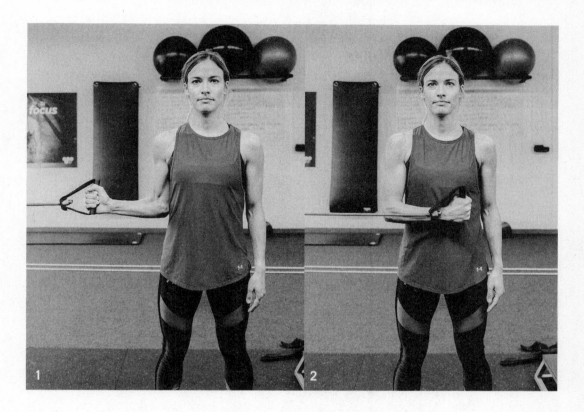

3 Next, remain standing with your right side facing the cable pulley station but move a step or two away from it and grasp the handle in your right hand. Begin with your right shoulder fully externally rotated (as in the finish position of the previous exercise) and tension on the cable.

4 Keeping your elbow and upper arm pressed against the side of your body, rotate your shoulder internally. Go all the way until your forearm is touching your belly button and return to the start position. Complete 10 repetitions with a weight you could lift 12 times with perfect form, then reverse your position and complete a set of internal shoulder rotations with your left arm.

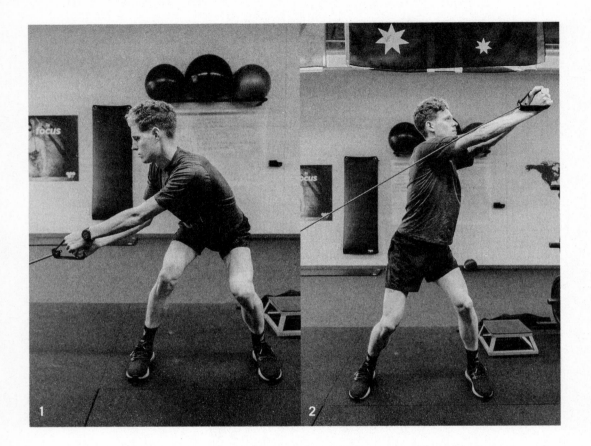

Standing Cable Low-High Pull

Lower back, upper back, shoulders

1 Connect a D-handle to a cable pulley station at ankle height. Stand in a wide stance with your left side facing the cable pulley station and most of your weight on the left foot. Grasp the handle in both hands, beginning with the handle just outside your knee.

2 Using both arms, pull the cable upward and across your body, keeping your arms straight and finishing with your hands above your right shoulder. Avoid rounding your back. Return smoothly to the start position. Complete 10 repetitions with a weight you could lift 12 times with perfect form, then reverse your position and repeat the exercise.

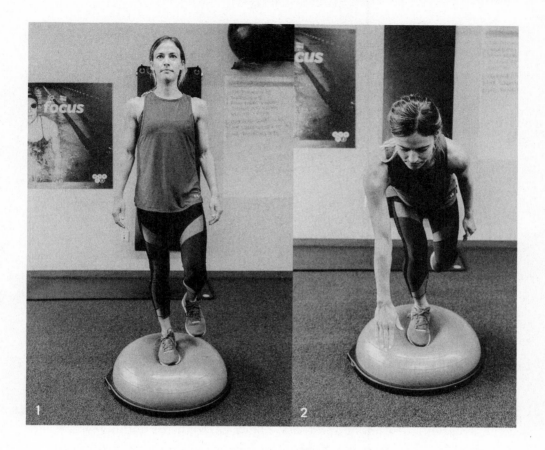

Single-Leg Balancing
Lower legs

1 Stand on a balance disk or BOSU ball on your left foot only with your left knee slightly bent. Remain in this position while counting to 30. If you lose balance and have to put your left foot down, just continue where you left off. Now balance on the left foot for 30 seconds.

2 If this exercise is too easy for you, replace it with a single-leg balancing bend and reach. While balancing on one foot, bend at the knees and hips and reach toward a spot on the floor in front of you with the same hand. Go as far as you can without losing your balance (it may not be very far) and return to the start position. Complete 10 repetitions with each leg.

Static Stretch Sequence

■ **Equipment need:**
Elastic strap

■ **Recommended frequency:**
Daily, if possible (ideally after a swim,
ride, or run, but throughout the day is okay as well)

The twelve stretches described in this section may be performed all together as a stand-alone flexibility routine, but there are a couple of reasons you might choose to do otherwise. One is that the primary rationale for including static stretching in your triathlon training is to prevent injury by restoring normal range of motion to joints. Thus, there is no need to perform static stretching involving muscles that are not abnormally limiting your range of motion at a particular joint.

A second reason for skipping certain stretches is that, according to research, it is necessary to stretch a muscle for at least three minutes per day to maximize the functional benefits. That's a lot of time, so you may want to devote the time you have available to those specific stretches you need most.

Note that almost all triathletes are tighter than they should be in the chest, hip flexors, hamstrings, calves, and Achilles tendons, and that a little stretching certainly is better than none and is never harmful, so there's nothing wrong with doing most or all of these twelve stretches daily for a minimum of thirty seconds apiece as indicated in the individual exercise descriptions.

If you do commit to stretching specific problem areas for the optimal three to five minutes a day, the good news is that you don't have to do it all at once. It's okay to do a little here, a little there, throughout the day until you've met this quota, though the ideal time to stretch is immediately after a swim, ride, or run, when the muscles are warm and loosened.

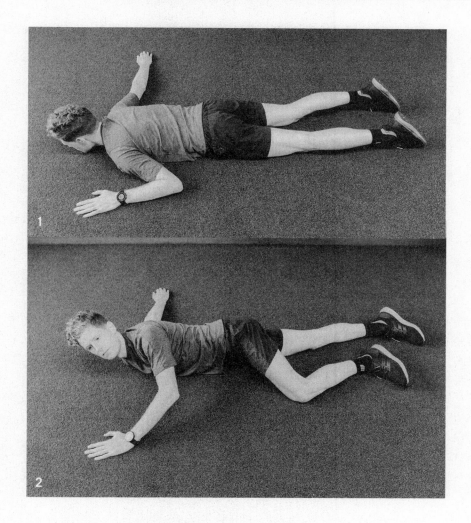

Chest and Front of Shoulder

1 Lie facedown and extend your right arm along the floor perpendicular to your body, palm down.

2 Press your left palm into the floor and rotate your entire body so that you come up onto your right side and you begin to feel a stretch in the right side of your chest, as well as in the front of your right shoulder. Hold the stretch for at least 30 seconds and then stretch your left side.

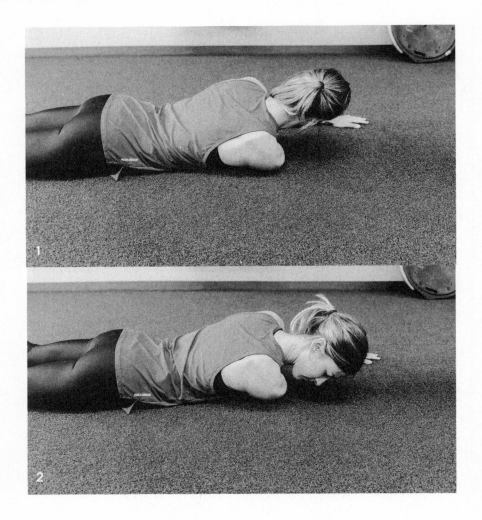

Back of Shoulder

1 Lie facedown with your right arm extended across your chest, palm up, and your weight on the upper arm.

2 Without moving that arm, twist your body slightly to the left until you feel a stretch in your right trapezium and rear deltoid. Hold it for at least 30 seconds and then reverse your position and stretch your left side.

Back and Triceps

Kneel on your hands and forearms and slide your forearms forward as far as possible while keeping your thighs perpendicular to the floor. Press your weight into your shoulder sockets and press your belly toward the floor. You'll feel a stretch in your lats and triceps. Hold it for 20 seconds, then roll slightly to the right for 20 seconds, and finally rotate to the left and hold for 20 seconds, for a total stretch time of 1 minute.

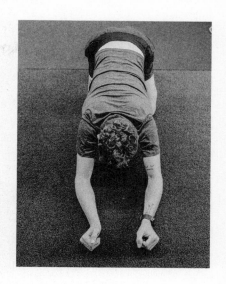

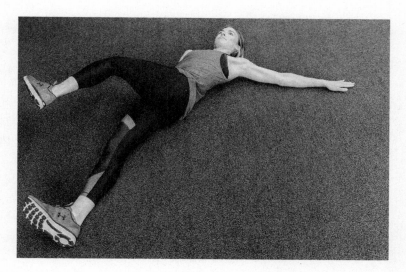

Glutes and Hip Abductors

Lie on your back with your left arm extended away from your body and resting palm-down on the floor. Bend your left leg 90 degrees and reach the knee across your body and toward the floor outside your right hip. Make sure your left shoulder blade remains in contact with the floor. Use pressure from your right hand to enhance the stretch. Hold it for at least 30 seconds and then stretch your right side.

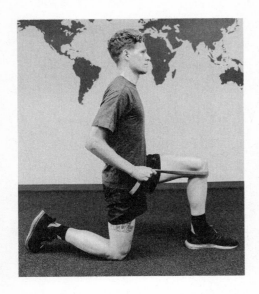

Hip Flexors

Kneel on your right knee and place your left foot flat on the floor with a 90-degree bend in the left knee. Grab the ends of a short strap in both hands, loop it around your left knee, and pull gently toward you. Keeping your torso upright, contract your glutes and press your hips forward until you feel a stretch at the front of your right hip. Hold the stretch for at least 30 seconds and then reverse your position and stretch the left hip.

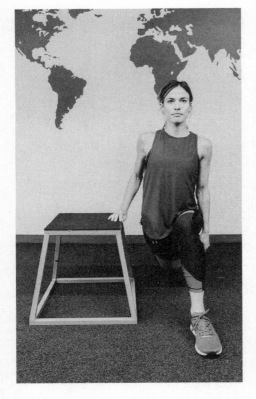

Tensor Fascia Lata (Outer Hip)

Kneel on your right knee and place your left foot flat on the floor with a 90-degree bend in the left knee and an exercise bench or some other stable platform to your immediate right. Shift your left foot slightly to the right so it's in line with your right knee. It may be difficult to balance in this position, so place the fingers of your right hand lightly on the exercise bench to keep from tipping (a wall will do if you don't have a bench).

To begin the stretch, tighten your right glute and press your right hip forward and to the right (toward the bench) while keeping the rest of your body completely stable. You should feel a stretch in the spot where the top of a jeans pocket would be if you were wearing them. Hold it for at least 30 seconds and then reverse your position and stretch the other hip.

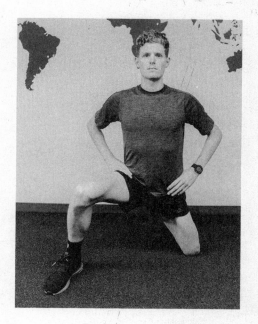

Hip Adductors

Perform this stretch just as you would the hip-flexor stretch, but without the strap and with your forward leg angled out 45 degrees, instead of straight ahead. Again, hold the stretch for at least 30 seconds and then stretch the opposite side.

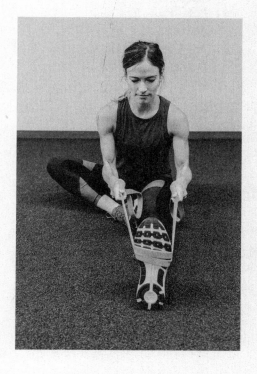

Hamstrings

Sit with your left leg outstretched in front of you and a strap looped around the foot with the ends held in your hands. Splay your right knee wide and tuck the foot against the inside of your left thigh. Bend forward from the hips and pull on the strap with just enough force to feel a stretch along the back of your left leg. Don't round your back; that'll increase your reach but take emphasis off your hamstrings, making the stretch less effective. Hold for at least 30 seconds and then stretch your right leg.

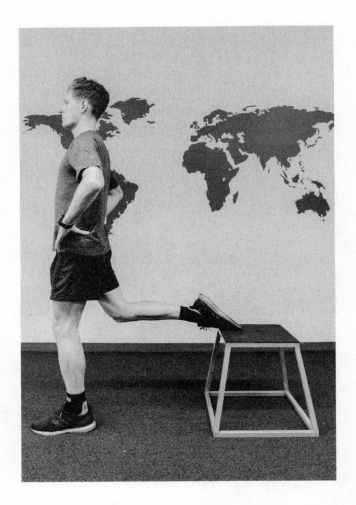

Quadriceps

Stand on your left foot and rest the top of the right foot on an exercise bench or similar platform, positioned so that your right thigh is perpendicular to the floor. Rest your hands on your hips. Rotate your pelvis backward and press your hips forward. You should feel a stretch along the front of the right thigh. Hold the stretch for 30 seconds and then stretch the left leg.

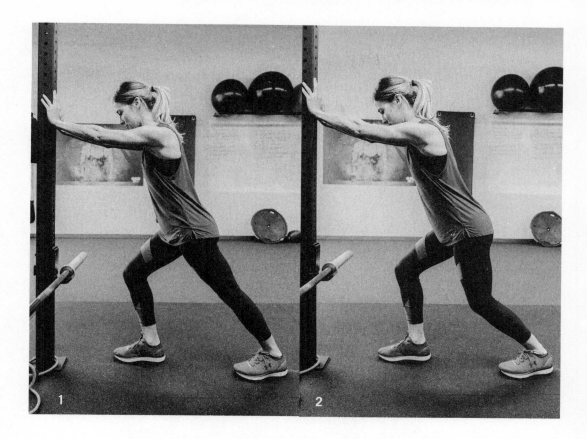

Gastrocnemius and Soleus

1 Brace your hands against a wall and extend your right leg far enough behind you that you feel a stretch in your calf when you place the foot flat on the ground. Hold the stretch for at least 30 seconds and then bend the knee slightly so that the stretch migrates deeper inside your calf.

2 Hold this stretch for at least 30 seconds and then stretch the left calf.

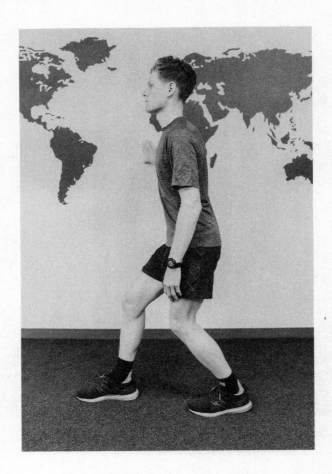

Achilles Tendon

Stand in a split stance, the left foot a step ahead of the right, with both feet flat on the ground and both knees slightly bent. Now bend your right leg a little more and concentrate on trying to "sink" your butt straight down toward the heel of that foot. Keep your torso upright. You should begin to feel a stretch in your Achilles tendon. You may have to fiddle with your position before you find it. When you do, hold it for at least 30 seconds, relax, and then stretch the opposite leg.

Mobility Exercise Sequence

■ **Equipment needed:** Broomstick

■ **Recommended frequency:** At least twice per week, as often as daily

The nine movements in this mobility exercise sequence should be done at least twice per week and may be done as often as daily. You can do them as a stand-alone session at any time, but there are other options. One is to do selected movements as part of your warm-ups for swims, bike rides, and runs. We recommend doing the wall ankle mobilization, the thoracic spine rotation, the dynamic chest stretch with broomstick, the scapular wall slide, and the wall circle before swims, as these movements mobilize joints emphasized in the water. The walking butt kick and supine hip stretch are good ones to do before hopping on the bike, and the remaining exercises—squat stretch and lunge walk with overheard reach—should be done before any run that entails efforts at or above Zone 3.

You may also fold together this exercise sequence with your strength workouts. Do this by alternating mobility movements with strength movements, preceding each strength movement with a mobility movement that targets the same part of the body, as in this example:

Mobility: Walking Butt Kick	Mobility: Thoracic Spine Rotation
Strength: Side Step-Up	Strength: Stability Ball Walk Out
Mobility: Lunge with Overhead Reach	Mobility: Wall Ankle Mobilization
Strength: Stick Crunch	Strength: Eccentric Heel Dip
Mobility: Dynamic Chest Stretch with Broomstick	Mobility: Supine Hip Rotation
Strength: Scapular Push-Up	Strength: Stability Ball Trunk Rotation
Mobility: Squat to Stand	Mobility: Wall Circle
Strength: Stability Ball Hamstrings Curl	Strength: Inverted Shoulder Press
Strength: Side Plank	Strength: Side Lying Hip Lift

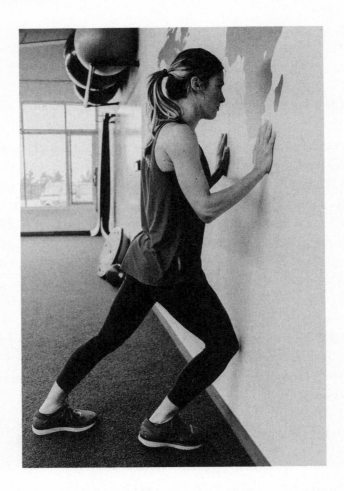

Wall Ankle Mobilization

Calves, Achilles tendons

This movement improves ankle mobility. Stand facing a wall, with the toes of the left foot against the wall, and bring the knee forward to tap the wall with your knee-cap. Straighten your knee and then slide the foot back a tiny bit so that your toes are about an inch away from the wall, and repeat. Keeping moving back little by little until you get to the exact point where the kneecap is *barely* touching the wall. Make sure that your knee goes straight forward and not inward, and that the heel remains on the floor the entire time. Perform 8 repetitions on each side.

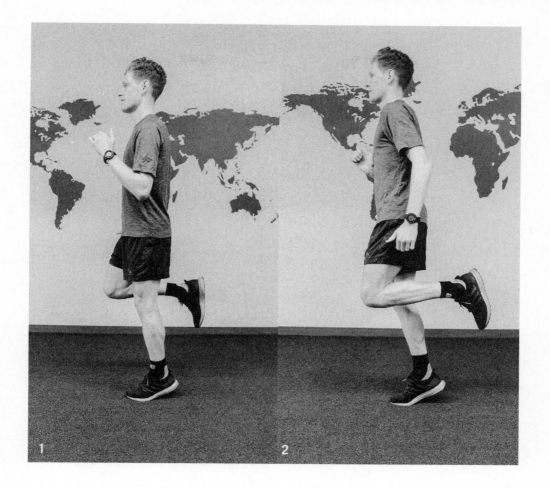

Walking Butt Kick

Quadriceps, hip flexors

1 From a standing position, take a step forward with the left leg and kick the heel of your right leg backward toward your glutes. Use your right hand to pull the heel into your glutes and come up on the toes of the opposite foot simultaneously. Maintain good posture (avoid forward leaning) and do not allow the leg to move to the side.

2 Hold this position for one second and then take a step with the right leg and stretch the left. Perform 5 repetitions with each leg.

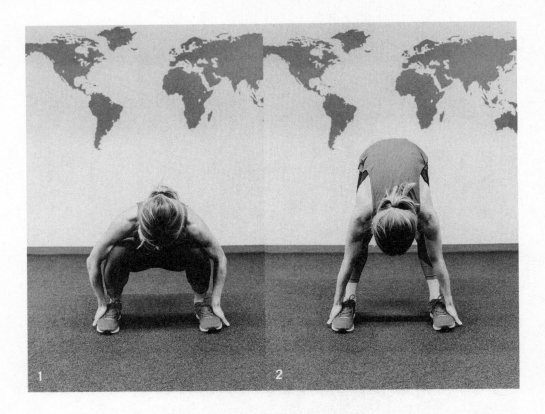

Squat to Stand

Hamstrings, groin

1 Stand with your feet positioned slightly farther than shoulder width apart. Bend over and grab the bottoms of your toes with your hands, bending your knees as much as necessary to do so. From here, use your arms to pull yourself into a deep squat position. Try to keep your chest up, your knees out, and a slight arch in your lower back.

2 Hold for 2 seconds before slowly extending your knees and raising your butt while keeping your hands under your feet. Complete 10 repetitions.

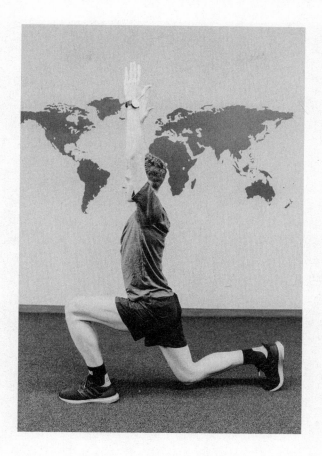

Lunge Walk with Overhead Reach
Hip flexors

Stand normally and raise both arms straight overhead. Take a long step forward with your left leg and bend both knees until your left thigh is parallel to the floor. Now thrust forward off the right foot and lunge with the left leg, keeping your arms raised. Perform 5 repetitions on each side.

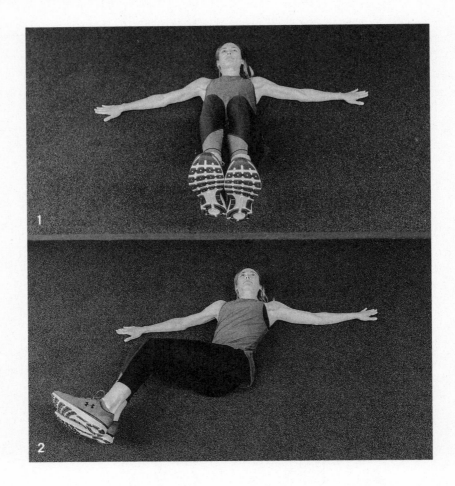

Supine Hip Rotation

Lower back

1 Lie face up on a comfortable surface. Bend your knees 90 degrees and elevate both legs so your thighs are pointing toward the ceiling. Spread your arms out away from your body along the floor, palms down.

2 Twist your hips to the right so your legs swing down toward the floor on that side. Go as far as you can without allowing your left shoulder blade to lose contact with the floor. Return to the start position and then twist to the left. Complete 8 repetitions on each side.

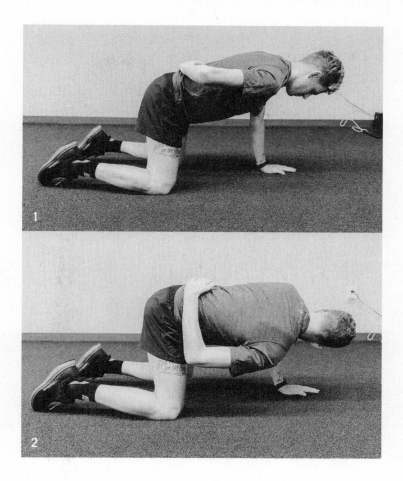

Thoracic Spine Rotation
Midback

1 Kneel on all fours. Lift and bend your right arm and rest the back of your hand against your lower spine.

2 Now twist your torso to the left so that your right elbow swivels toward your left arm, which should be kept straight. Now rotate back toward the start position, but go a bit farther, so that your eyes are directed toward the wall to your right. Complete 10 rotations and then reverse your arm positions and rotate the opposite way.

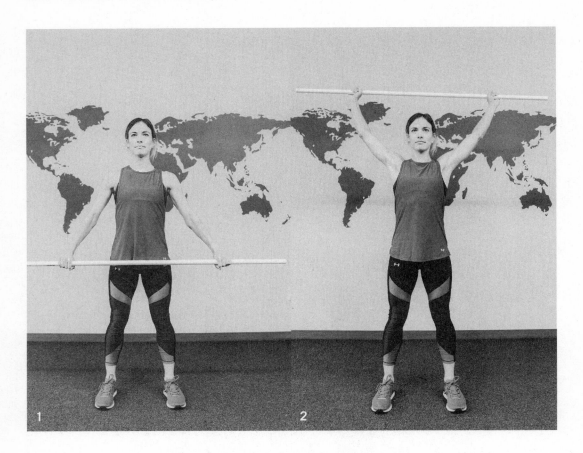

Dynamic Chest Stretch with Broomstick
Chest, shoulders, upper back

1 Stand normally while grasping a broomstick or similar object near both ends in an overhand grip. Begin with the broomstick resting against your thighs.

2 Now raise the broomstick up overhead and back as if you're trying to pass it to someone standing behind you. When you've reached the end of your range of motion, squeeze your rear shoulders in an effort to press the broomstick just a little farther back and then return to the start position. Repeat at total of 6 times.

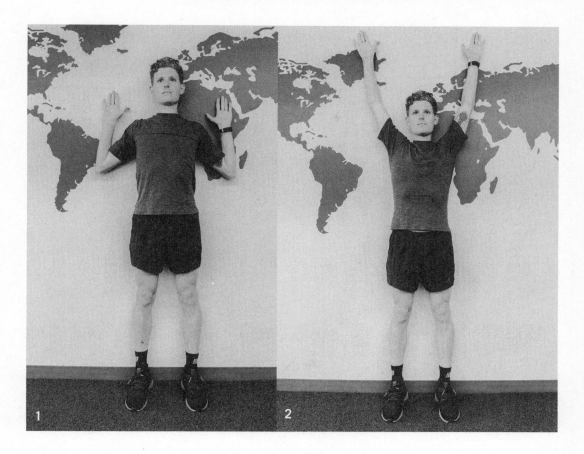

Scapular Wall Slide

Shoulders

1 Stand with your butt, upper back, and head pressed against a wall. Bend your elbows sharply and press both arms into the wall with the palms of your hands facing forward. Begin with your elbows tucked close to your sides and your hands at approximately shoulder level.

2 Now slide your arms slowly upward against the wall until you look like a football referee signaling a touchdown. Keep your butt, back, shoulder blades, head, elbows, and the backs of your hands pressed against the wall the whole way. Now slowly return to the start position. Repeat this sliding movement 6 times.

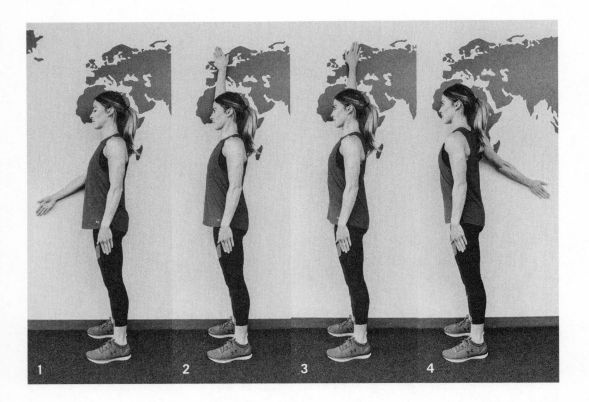

Wall Circle

Shoulders

1 Stand with your right side against a wall and your right arm extended downward, palm facing you.

2 Slowly raise your arm, tracing a circle on the wall with your fingernails.

3–4 Continue until you reach the limit of your range of motion, then flip your hand around so the palm is against the wall and complete the circle by rotating your arm back and behind your body until it is once again between your body and the wall. Now reverse your position and draw a wall circle with your left arm.

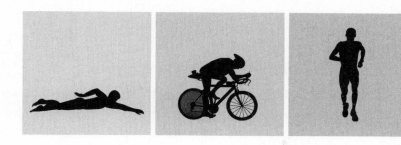

8

Getting Started with 80/20 Training

Effective triathlon training requires planning. Whether you're new to the sport or you're a seasoned age-group awards chaser, you will achieve greater improvements in fitness and performance if you follow a well-designed training plan than if you wing it. Creating a triathlon training plan is not rocket science (trust us: we do it every day, and we're not rocket scientists!), but it does require an understanding of not only the 80/20 Rule of intensity balance but of other proven training principles and practices as well.

Only a small fraction of triathletes choose to create their own training plans, the rest preferring to leave this job to the experts. You may share this preference, in which case you will want to start your 80/20 triathlon journey by following one of the ready-made plans you'll find in the next few chapters. But even if you do, you will still benefit from learning the principles and best practices of training plan design, as it will help you make good decisions when you need to modify or depart from your plan due to fatigue, soreness, or other factors, and it will give you the option to begin coaching yourself down the road.

While the 80/20 approach provides a simple guideline for balancing the intensity of training, there's a bit more to the process of creating an effective triathlon training program. In this chapter we will walk you through the six steps of creating your own custom 80/20 triathlon training plan.

Step 1: Define your training cycle.

A training cycle is a multiweek period of progressive training that begins when you embark on the process of building fitness for competition and ends with either a single important race (or "A" race) or with the first race in a series. Training plans should line up with training cycles, beginning and ending at the same points.

The appropriate length of a training cycle/plan is twelve to twenty-four weeks. Triathletes who try to build fitness for periods exceeding twenty-four weeks tend to burn out, become injured, or lose motivation. So, if your next race is many months away, you should wait until it's twenty-four weeks out or less before you begin a formal ramp-up for that event and in the meantime do maintenance training. Regardless of the duration of your training plan, you should take a break to allow your body to regenerate after you've completed it. The ideal time to start a new training plan is after such a break. Because your fitness level will be well below the preceding peak at this time, you will need to allow at least twelve weeks to prepare for your next race—hence our recommended minimum duration for triathlon training plans.

Whether the plan you design for yourself is closer to twelve or twenty-four weeks in length should depend on a few factors. The fitter you are or expect to be at the start of the cycle, the less time it will take you to attain peak fitness. Additionally, training cycle lengths should be proportional to the distance of your A race. The longer your race is, the more time you'll need to allow regardless of your initial fitness level. Ironman training plans will creep toward twenty-four weeks, sprint plans hew closer to twelve.

Another consideration is the number of races you intend to do. There are two general approaches to triathlon competition. Some athletes like to prepare for a single "A" race, including no more than one or two lower-priority triathlons (or "B" races) in the lead-up to it. This approach is widely preferred by those who are focused on longer events, which, by their very nature, cannot be contested frequently. Other athletes like to take a seasonal approach to the sport, doing a number of shorter races (usually sprints and/or Olympic-distance events, with perhaps the occasional half Ironman thrown in) within a relatively short span of time.

The seasonal approach makes for trickier planning due to the disruptive effect that racing has on training. More stressful than any workout, races require you to rest both before you do them (so you're not fatigued before you even start) and after you do them (so the fatigue acquired during the race doesn't wreak havoc on your subsequent training). For this reason, it is virtually impossible to build fitness while racing often.

You can minimize the disruptiveness of the seasonal approach by making a distinction between the *training cycle* and the *racing cycle*. A racing cycle is a period of frequent racing that comes immediately after the training cycle, where the goal is not to gain additional fitness but to take advantage of fitness gained already and race repeatedly at close to top form. The key to a successful racing cycle is training very lightly between events. This limits the risk of injury and burnout even if the combined duration of the training and racing cycles exceeds twenty-four weeks. For example, a 16-week training cycle in which you train 90 minutes a day on average and do not compete at all might be followed by a 10-week racing cycle in which you race six or eight times and train less than 60 minutes a day between sprint or Olympic-distance triathlons.

The disadvantage of tacking a multiweek racing cycle onto a training cycle is that, because the training volume is necessarily low, no new fitness can be gained, and performance will gradually erode. For this reason, racing cycles themselves should seldom exceed ten or twelve weeks. It's true that professional triathletes who compete on the ITU World Cup circuit routinely engage in racing seasons that stretch from March all the way to September, but they do not train progressively for this entire six-month period. Instead, they insert one or more regeneration periods at crucial points to ensure they don't overcook themselves. Follow their example if your race schedule looks similar to that of the typical short-course pro.

When you've decided on the start and end dates of your training cycle (and possibly also your separate racing cycle) and chosen all of the races you wish to do in this period, schedule these events on your calendar. By way of illustrating the training plan design process, we will create a plan for a hypothetical triathlete named Laura. Given that the ready-made training plans presented in the next four chapters do a thorough job of demonstrating what a training cycle targeting a single "A" race should look like, we'll make Laura a seasonal type of triathlete who likes to do several shorter events each summer. Laura sets the start date of her plan to fall eight weeks before her first race, a sprint, to give herself time to build fitness throughout the spring, following a winter of lighter training. Because Laura likes to compete often, she squeezes four more races into the next sixteen weeks, the most she can reasonably expect to do without creating the need for a separate racing cycle. The training cycle ends on the day of the last race, making the full cycle twenty-four weeks in length.

Table 8.1 shows what Laura's schedule looks like after Step 1 of the training plan design process. The shading you see in certain rows will be explained in the next section.

TABLE 8.1
**An Example of a Custom
80/20 Triathlon Training Plan After Step 1**

WEEK	MON	TUE	WED	THU	FRI	SAT	SUN
1							
2							
3							
4							
5							
6							
7							
8						Sprint	
9							
10						Olympic	
11							
12							
13							
14							
15							Olympic
16							
17							
18							
19						Sprint	
20							
21							
22							
23							
24							Olympic

Step 2: Schedule recovery weeks.

To finish a training cycle fitter than you were at the beginning, you need to increase your training load (which factors together both volume and intensity) gradually throughout it. For example, your training load in Week 16 should be somewhat greater than your training load in Week 6. Your workouts should not become more challenging every single week, however. Instead, you'll want to designate every third or fourth week as a recovery week, where the training load is actually reduced. The reason is simple: If you try to increase your training load every week, you will become more and more fatigued until exhaustion or injury forces you to take a break. Giving your body a chance to catch up on rest periodically over the course of a training cycle will enable you to handle heavier training loads and attain a higher fitness level by the end.

Recovery weeks come at the end of step cycles, which are three- to four-week blocks of training in which each week is slightly more challenging than the one before until the last week of the block, which is a recovery week. Any and all races included in your training cycle should fall at the end of a step cycle—that is, at the end of a recovery week—to ensure that your body is fresh and ready for the stress of competition. It is for this reason that scheduling recovery weeks is the logical next step in the process of building a training plan. But it's not only race weeks that should be designated as recovery weeks. You should set aside every third or fourth week for recovery even during periods when you're not racing.

Plan to reduce your total training hours by 30 to 40 percent in each recovery week relative to the preceding week, a 30 percent reduction being adequate during lighter periods of training and a 40 percent reduction necessary during heavier periods. Three-week step cycles typically work best for beginner and older athletes and during very intensive periods of training. Four-week step cycles are preferable during lighter periods of training, for athletes who train relatively lightly in general, and for advanced athletes willing and able to train hard for three straight weeks before resting.

If you're lucky, your scheduled races will line up perfectly with your step cycles, always coinciding with weeks that would have been recovery weeks anyway. For example, if you are planning a twenty-week training cycle with four-week step cycles, the ideal times for races would be Week 12, Week 16, and Week 20. But things seldom work out quite so neatly, and when they don't, it becomes necessary to make some judgment calls on where to place recovery opportunities.

Two tools that are helpful in these situations are half recovery weeks and semirecovery weeks. A half recovery week is one in which an athlete trains normally for either the first few days or the last few days and trains less on the other days. A semirecovery week is one in which the training load is reduced throughout, but by less than 30 percent.

Laura's training plan has a use for both of these tools. Notice in Table 8.2 that she has a pair of races just fourteen days apart in Weeks 8 and 10. If she treats both of these weeks as normal recovery weeks, she risks getting too much rest and not enough quality training during this period. She can minimize this issue, however, by making Week 10 a half recovery week, training normally in the first few days and then reducing her workload in the last few days before her race.

Later in the training cycle, Laura faces a somewhat different challenge. If she begins a new four-week step cycle after her Week 10 race, then Week 14 will be her next recovery week. But Week 15 contains another race, and it is therefore already designated as a recovery week. It doesn't make much sense to schedule back-to-back recovery weeks. Laura could avoid this issue by treating Weeks 11 through 15 as an extended, five-week step cycle, but that would be risky. Few athletes can survive four straight weeks of progressive training without digging a hole for themselves. The best way for Laura to balance her needs for quality training and for recovery during this period is to treat Week 13 as a semirecovery week, in which the training load is reduced, but by less than the usual 30 to 40 percent.

Recovery weeks that precede important races are referred to as a taper. A one- or two-week taper is usually sufficient for athletes who train relatively lightly. The heavier the peak training load is, the longer the taper should be. Elite triathletes often taper for three full weeks before a longer race, reducing their training load modestly in the first week (in other words, treating it as a semirecovery week) and dialing back a little more each week thereafter. Laura intends her peak training volume to be moderately high, so she plans a two-week, two-step taper.

Table 8.2 shows Laura's training plan with recovery and taper weeks added (refer to Appendices A, B, and C to decode the specific workouts selected). Darker shading indicates a full recovery week, lighter shading a semirecovery week.

TABLE 8.2

Example Training Plan with Recovery and Taper Weeks Added

WEEK	SPORT	MON	TUE	WED	THU	FRI	SAT	SUN	WEEKLY DISTANCE/ DURATION	
1	Swim									
	Cycle									
	Run									
2	Swim									
	Cycle									
	Run									
3	Swim									
	Cycle									
	Run									
4	Swim			STT2		SF2		SCI1	4100	
	Cycle			CF3	CT29			CFF27	2:25	5:36
	Run		RF8				RCI1		1:55	
5	Swim									
	Cycle									
	Run									
6	Swim									
	Cycle									
	Run									
7	Swim									
	Cycle									
	Run									
8	Swim			STT2		SF4			3000	
	Cycle			CF3	CF9		Sprint		1:30	4:55
	Run		RF10						2:30	
9	Swim									
	Cycle									
	Run									
10	Swim			STT2		SF3			2750	
	Cycle			CF9	CF5		Olympic		1:40	6:05
	Run		RF8						3:35	

(continues)

(continued)

TABLE 8.2
Example Training Plan with Recovery and Taper Weeks Added

WEEK	SPORT	MON	TUE	WED	THU	FRI	SAT	SUN	WEEKLY DISTANCE/ DURATION	
11	Swim									
	Cycle									
	Run									
12	Swim									
	Cycle									
	Run									
13	Swim			STT2			SCI2	SF1	4500	6:28
	Cycle			CT29	CF5			CCI13	3:05	
	Run		RF10			RT11			2:00	
14	Swim									
	Cycle								3:40	
	Run								3:00	
15	Swim			STT2			SCI2		3000	6:25
	Cycle			CF9		CF5		Olympic	1:40	
	Run		RF10						3:50	
16	Swim									
	Cycle									
	Run									
17	Swim									
	Cycle									
	Run									
18	Swim									
	Cycle									
	Run									
19	Swim			STT2					3000	6:00
	Cycle			CT30		CF3	Sprint		1:30	
	Run		RF12		RF6				3:35	
20	Swim									
	Cycle									
	Run									

TABLE 8.2
Example Training Plan with Recovery and Taper Weeks Added

WEEK	SPORT	MON	TUE	WED	THU	FRI	SAT	SUN	WEEKLY DISTANCE/ DURATION	
21	Swim									
	Cycle									
	Run									
22	Swim									
	Cycle									
	Run									
23	Swim		SCI12		SAe1			SF1	6500	
	Cycle			CCI19			CF10	BR3	3:00	8:14
	Run		RF6			RF12			2:15	
24	Swim			SSI1		SCI1	STa1		4250	
	Cycle		CF9		CCI17		CRe1	Olympic	1:50	6:58
	Run		RCI13		RF3		RTa1		3:50	

Step 3: Create a default weekly workout schedule (or microcycle).

The basic building blocks of a training cycle are microcycles, or recurring sequences of swim, bike, and run workouts. For practical reasons, microcycles are almost always one week in length. With a seven-day rotation, it's easy to ensure that the most time-consuming workouts always fall on Saturday and Sunday, or whenever your days off from work or school happen to be. We recommend that you employ one-week microcycles unless you have a compelling reason to do otherwise.

Having established the length of your microcycles, you next need to decide how many times per week you wish to swim, ride, and run, and how to distribute these sessions throughout the week. Regardless of your level of experience in each discipline, we suggest that you consider two swims, two rides, and two runs per week as a minimum frequency. It's difficult to make much progress as a triathlete if you don't exercise almost every day. Six total workouts per week are plenty for most beginners, but if you've already reached the point where you've gotten as much improvement as you can get from this schedule (for example by increasing the challenge level of the harder sessions to a reasonable limit), you will need to add more workouts to your microcycle to stimulate further gains. It's important that you do this gradually, adding one new session at a time.

In general, your microcycles should include equal or nearly equal numbers of workouts in each discipline. So, for example, if your microcycle contains nine workouts, the breakdown should be three swims, three rides, and three runs, not two swims, five rides, and two runs. If you are already doing equal numbers of swims, rides, and runs, and you wish to add workouts to your microcycle, we recommend that you do so in either (a) descending order of the impact that each discipline has on overall triathlon performance, inserting a bike ride first, a run second, and a swim last; or (b) ascending order of your personal strength in each discipline (e.g., adding a swim first if swimming is your weakest discipline). The first option will tend to maximize performance in imminent races, whereas the second can turn weaknesses into strengths over time and may yield better overall triathlon performance in the long term.

Although it is generally true that the more frequently you train, the fitter you will become, there is a law of diminishing returns. Going from two sessions per discipline per week to three will have a greater impact than going from three to four. So, don't feel compelled to keep adding workouts to your schedule in search of progress. There are other ways to improve, such as lengthening the workouts you're already doing.

Many athletes are limited not by how many workouts their body can handle but by how many their schedule can accommodate. Time constraints aside, your workout frequency should be determined by your training history (again, your workout frequency or duration in any given training cycle should never be more than slightly greater than it was in the last one), your level of competitiveness (the more ambitious your race goals are, the more worthwhile it may be to increase your workout frequency in pursuit of small gains), and the length of your next race (it's a lot easier to get by on six total workouts per week if you're preparing for a sprint than if you're ramping up for an Ironman).

Table 8.3 summarizes our recommended weekly workout frequency progression. The idea is to start with the workout numbers in the first row if you're a beginner and then advance gradually through the subsequent rows, stopping when you are doing as much training as your schedule can accommodate or your

TABLE 8.3
Recommended Weekly Workout Frequency Progression

ATHLETE TYPE	SWIMS	BIKE RIDES	RUNS
Beginner	2	2	2
	2	3	2
	2	3	3
	3	3	3
	3	4	3
Highly Experienced and Competitive	3	4	4
	4	4	4

body can handle. We consider this a good blueprint for most triathletes, but it's not the only way to go. To return to an earlier example, if you are an especially weak swimmer, you may want to swim more often than you ride and run until you've gotten stronger in the water.

Once you've settled on the number of workouts you wish to include in your microcycles, your next move is to decide when to do them. The objective is to distribute workouts in each discipline as evenly as possible throughout the week. For example, if you plan to swim three times per week, don't schedule these workouts on Monday, Tuesday, and Wednesday, and then go four days without swimming.

Workouts should be distributed across the week not only by sport discipline but also on the basis of workout format. Within each discipline, there are four basic categories of workout: (a) easy swims, rides, and runs (i.e., relatively short sessions done in Zone 1 and/or 2); (b) long endurance-building workouts; (c) moderate-intensity swims, rides, and runs (i.e., sessions focused on either Zone X or Zone 3); and (d) high-intensity interval workouts (i.e., sessions focused on Zone 4 and/or Zone 5). It's best to avoid scheduling workouts of the same type close together. For example, although there's nothing wrong with riding your bike and running on the same day, try not to schedule a high-intensity ride and a high-intensity run on the same day.

An exception to this principle must often be made, however, for long endurance workouts. Most triathletes have no choice but to do their long endurance rides and runs on the weekend because these workouts take a long time and are difficult or impossible to squeeze into workdays or schooldays.

The three tables following offer possible ways of distributing workouts by discipline and format throughout a seven-day microcycle. Table 8.3 is relevant to athletes who train twice per week in each discipline, Table 8.4 is for those who do three swims, three rides, and three runs per microcycle, and Table 8.5 applies to athletes who train four times per week in each discipline.

If you train less than four times per week in each discipline, you will not be able to do swims, rides, and runs of all four formats in any single week. This isn't a problem. All that matters is that whatever combination of workouts you include in a given week allows you to apply the 80/20 Rule when you fill in the calendar with specific workouts. In this regard, keep in mind that moderate- and high-intensity workouts are not performed *exclusively* at these intensities but include some work at low intensity. This makes it feasible to consistently do 80 percent of your weekly training at low intensity regardless of your training frequency and despite including a moderate- or high-intensity workout in each discipline in your microcycle. All three of our suggested microcycles are conducive to maintaining an 80/20 intensity balance when coupled with the workouts in Appendices A, B, and C.

The purpose of creating a default weekly workout schedule is not to lock yourself into repeating the same pattern over and over throughout the entire training cycle (for example *always* doing a high-intensity run on Tuesday). Your microcycle may need to evolve somewhat as you schedule specific sessions for each week and consider how they impact and are impacted by other sessions. If you study the ready-made training plans in Chapters 10 through 14, you will see that workout categories tend to float around somewhat from week to week. For example, you may be asked to perform a high-intensity interval run on Tuesday in Week 4 and on Thursday the following week. Such shifting is an outcome of the many factors we considered in designing the plans. Don't lose sleep over this. By analyzing our plans, you will observe patterns that you can incorporate into the training plans you make for yourself, and in the meantime, the simple patterns represented in the following tables provide a solid starting point.

Laura, our hypothetical triathlete, has a few years of experience under her belt and is fairly competitive, but she also has a busy life outside of her sport and she tends to get run down when she's too aggressive with her training. Most triathletes who fit this description feel comfortable with a seven-day microcycle that includes three swims, three rides, and three runs, and that's true of Laura as well. Therefore she will use a microcycle similar to the one in Table 8.5.

TABLE 8.4

Sample Weekly Training Schedule by Workout Category for Triathletes Who Train 6 Times per Week

MONDAY	TUESDAY	WEDNESDAY	THURSDAY	FRIDAY	SATURDAY	SUNDAY
Rest	High-Intensity Run	Endurance Swim or Moderate-Intensity Swim	High-Intensity Bike	High-Intensity Swim	Endurance Run or Moderate-Intensity Run	Endurance Bike or Moderate-Intensity Bike

TABLE 8.5

Sample Weekly Training Schedule by Workout Category for Triathletes Who Train 9 Times per Week

MONDAY	TUESDAY	WEDNESDAY	THURSDAY	FRIDAY	SATURDAY	SUNDAY
Rest	High-Intensity Swim	High-Intensity Bike	Moderate-Intensity Swim	Endurance Swim	Endurance Run	Endurance Bike (or Brick)
	Moderate-Intensity Run		High-Intensity Run	Moderate-Intensity Bike		

TABLE 8.6

Sample Weekly Training Schedule by Workout Category for Triathletes Who Train 12 Times per Week

MONDAY	TUESDAY	WEDNESDAY	THURSDAY	FRIDAY	SATURDAY	SUNDAY
High-Intensity Swim*	Easy Bike	Endurance Swim	Moderate-Intensity Swim	Moderate-Intensity Bike	Endurance Run	Endurance Swim
	Moderate-Intensity Run	High-Intensity Bike	High-Intensity Run	Easy Run		Endurance Bike (or Brick)

*This swim can be moved to Saturday to allow for a full day off.

Step 4: Plan your peak training step cycle.

When you take a long road trip in your car, you need to know your final destination before you can decide which way to turn at the end of your driveway. Similarly, the proper starting point of a training plan is actually the endpoint. Before you can make sensible decisions about how to train in the beginning and middle of a training cycle, you need to know where it's going. Specifically, you need to plan your peak step cycle, which is your heaviest two to three weeks of training featuring your most challenging individual workouts. The purpose of the peak step cycle is to put the final touches on your race readiness, and it should fall right before you begin your final taper.

The purpose of each preceding step cycle is to prepare you for the next one. The peak step cycle therefore acts as a benchmark that enables you to plan a sensible progression in workload across the span of step cycles that make up your training plan. For example, if you are able to commit to a maximum of ten hours of training in Week 18, you will not want to start out with nine hours in Week 1. Something closer to six hours would allow for a natural progression through the step cycles to your upper limit of ten hours.

In planning your peak step cycle, select workouts that simulate the endurance and speed challenges of your upcoming race. We strongly recommend that, instead of creating workouts from scratch, you draw from the pool of swim, bike, run, and brick workouts presented in the appendices. Choose workouts that would be too hard for you to handle today but that you can realistically expect to be able to handle when the time comes.

Not all the workouts in your peak step cycle should be difficult, though. The centerpiece of your peak step cycle will be race-specific workouts in each discipline. Any other workouts included in this period should serve as fitness maintainers, not fitness builders. Yet even these workouts may be longer than the sessions serving the same purpose that you do early in the training cycle.

If you've never written your own training plan before, you may have no clue where to begin. In this case, we suggest you use the peak step cycles in our ready-made 80/20 triathlon plans as templates. (Note that they do not fall at the same point in every plan. To identify them, look for the last two to three weeks of heavy volume preceding an obvious taper.) You will find the following key principles exemplified in them. Incorporate the same principles in planning your peak training step cycle.

- 80 percent of your total planned swimming, cycling, and running time is in Zones 1 and 2. (See the sidebar on page 138 for guidelines on how to plan 80/20 training weeks.)

- Most of the remaining 20 percent of your planned swimming, cycling, and running time is performed in Zone 3 (this zone being closer to race intensity than Zones 4 and 5, which should be prioritized earlier in the training cycle).

- The overall volume of training (i.e., total combined swimming, cycling, and running time/distance) is close to, but slightly less than, the maximum volume you anticipate being able to handle at this point in your training.

- The single most challenging workout of the peak step cycle is a weekly bike-run brick workout. In half and full Ironman training, this workout should be quite long and should take place mostly in Zone 2 to low Zone X. In training for all shorter distances, this brick workout should focus on Zone 3. Be sure to factor any time in Zone X into your 20 percent allotment of moderate to high intensity.

If you take a seasonal approach to the sport, doing a number of shorter races in each training cycle, as our hypothetical athlete Laura does (or in a separate racing cycle), you may want to include two peak step cycles in your plan, scheduling one before your final "A" race and the other before an earlier "A" race. This will allow you to perform at or near the same, maximal level in both of these events. Adding a third peak step cycle to your schedule will not enable you to do a third race at your highest level; rather, it will cause you to burn out. If you intend to do more than two races, you'll need to designate one or more of them as "B" races, forgo a preceding taper, and be content to do them at a fitness level that's a step or two below your peak. Laura has chosen to include two peak step cycles in her plan. Table 8.7 shows the plan with peak training step cycles added.

HOW TO PLAN AN 80/20 TRAINING WEEK

It's easy to plan a week of training that adheres to the 80/20 Rule if you use the preformatted workouts from Appendices A, B, and C. Each individual workout description includes information on time spent in each zone. After choosing your workouts for the week, divide the total weekly duration at low intensity (Zones 1 and 2) by the total weekly duration of all workouts. That result should be close to 80 percent.

There are a few nuances to consider, however. Because all 80/20 swim workouts are specified in distance, you will have to do a separate, distance-based calculation for this discipline. Additionally, if you're aiming to spend 80 percent of your total swim *time* at low intensity in a given week, you must plan to do 75 percent of your swim *distance* at low intensity. The reason is that you will cover more distance in less time when swimming in Zones 3–5. It is our experience that planning a swim week using a 75/25 distance-based distribution results in an 80/20 distribution in time. A more precise alternative is to meticulously track your actual time spent in each zone for the week and use this data to fine-tune subsequent swim planning. In our opinion, this is more work than it is worth.

Another consideration is how to handle Zone X. Recall that this zone counts as moderate intensity, so any time you spend in it counts toward the 20 side of the 80/20 ratio. Recall also that none of the 80/20 workouts prescribes Zone X, yet a few of them allow advanced athletes to spend time in this zone. If you intend to take advantage of this license, you will need to manually convert some of the Zone 2 workout time to Zone X and count it toward total planned time at moderate to high intensity for the week in which that workout falls.

For example, suppose you wish to include the cycling workout CAe10 in your schedule (5 min Z1, 5 × [30 min Z2/10 min Z1], 5 min Z1), and because you are very fit and experienced on the bike, you intend to accept our permission for athletes like you to do the Zone 2 intervals in Zone X. In this case, the workout shifts from 210 minutes at low intensity and 0 minutes at moderate/high intensity to 60 minutes at low intensity and 150 minutes at moderate intensity. Another option is to create your own custom workout that explicitly includes work in Zone X. As long as you exclude planned time in Zone X from your total weekly time at low intensity, you can utilize Zone X and still plan a week with the proper 80/20 distribution. Note that Zone Y does not merit consideration, as there is no scenario in which planning Zone Y in advance is recommended and in any case it falls between zones that already count toward the 20 side of 80/20.

Let's walk through the process using Laura's custom plan in Table 8.9. Week 11 includes three swims represented by workouts SMI1, SAe7, and SSP5. From Appendix A we find that these three workouts equal 5,250 total yards (or meters) of swimming, of which 4,000 yards are at low intensity (Zones 1 and 2) with the balance at moderate and high intensities. To calculate the intensity distribution of this week of swim training, Laura simply divides the total distance at low intensity by the total distance of all swim workouts, or 4,000 / 5,250 = 76 percent, which is very close to the 75/25 target.

The calculation for cycling and running is almost identical, but we will use duration instead of distance and the standard 80/20 target. Laura's Week 11 includes three bike rides—CCI1, CF6, and a CCI19—and three runs: RF3, RCI1, and an RF12. Appendices B and C inform us that the total duration of these bike and run workouts is 405 minutes, with 330 minutes at low intensity. Dividing 330 minutes by 405 minutes, we learn that 81 percent of the planned bike and run training for this week are at low intensity.

Your first attempt at validating the 80/20 ratios won't be this easy. It can take a few tries to find the right combination of workouts that conforms to the 80/20 Rule. Fortunately, the preformatted plans provided in Chapters 10 through 14 will give you hundreds of weeks of examples that already adhere to the 80/20 ratio. And bear in mind that there is no magic in round numbers. Ratios between 78/22 and 82/18 are close enough.

Nor will a single week of training that strays farther from the 80/20 ideal harm you if the step cycle of which it is a part obeys the 80/20 Rule. But it's best if every week is equally close to the mark, except during periods when you are intentionally aiming for a different balance; for example, when you are coming back from an injury and not yet ready for much work at high intensity.

Don't be alarmed if you notice that the intensity distributions of some of the 80/20 workouts in the appendices, particularly those including moderate- and high-intensity intervals, don't add up the way you would expect. In most cases, this is because short recovery intervals of less than 3 minutes are included in the time spent at moderate and high intensities (Zones 3–5). Our reason for this bit of fudging is that the stress of each hard interval continues to tax your body while you recover from it, so that counting the entire interval block, encompassing hard efforts and recoveries, as work at moderate or high intensity most accurately reflects the workout's physiological impact.

TABLE 8.7
Example Training Plan with Peak Training Weeks Added

WEEK	SPORT	MON	TUE	WED	THU	FRI	SAT	SUN	WEEKLY DISTANCE/ DURATION	
1	Swim									
	Cycle									
	Run									
2	Swim									
	Cycle									
	Run									
3	Swim									
	Cycle									
	Run									
4	Swim			STT2		SF2		SCI1	4100	
	Cycle			CF3	CT29			CFF27	2:25	5:36
	Run		RF8			RCI1			1:55	
5	Swim									
	Cycle									
	Run									
6	Swim									
	Cycle									
	Run									
7	Swim									
	Cycle									
	Run									
8	Swim			STT2		SF4			3000	
	Cycle			CF3	CF9		Sprint		1:30	4:55
	Run		RF10						2:30	
9	Swim									
	Cycle									
	Run									
10	Swim			STT2		SF3			2750	
	Cycle			CF9	CF5		Olympic		1:40	6:05
	Run		RF8						3:35	

TABLE 8.7
Example Training Plan with Peak Training Weeks Added

WEEK	SPORT	MON	TUE	WED	THU	FRI	SAT	SUN	WEEKLY DISTANCE/DURATION	
11	Swim									
	Cycle									
	Run									
12	Swim			SCI17		SAe1		SSI1	5750	
	Cycle			CF11	CAn1		CF13	BR3	4:30	8:51
	Run		RCI2			RRe6			2:37	
13	Swim			STT2			SCI2	SF1	4500	
	Cycle			CT29	CF5			CCI13	3:05	6:28
	Run		RF10			RT11			2:00	
14	Swim			SMI1		SAe7		SSP5	5250	
	Cycle		CF8	CF6	BR4			CF13	3:40	8:16
	Run		RF3				RF9		3:00	
15	Swim			STT2			SCI2		3000	
	Cycle			CF9	CF5			Olympic	1:40	6:25
	Run		RF10						3:50	
16	Swim									
	Cycle									
	Run									
17	Swim									
	Cycle									
	Run									
18	Swim									
	Cycle									
	Run									
19	Swim			STT2					3000	
	Cycle			CT30		CF3	Sprint		1:30	6:00
	Run		RF12		RF6				3:35	
20	Swim			SCI1		SAe1		SCI5	6000	
	Cycle		CCI5	CF6				CAe36	4:19	9:25
	Run		RF3		RAe6		RCI12		3:16	

(continues)

(continued)

TABLE 8.7

Example Training Plan with Peak Training Weeks Added

WEEK	SPORT	MON	TUE	WED	THU	FRI	SAT	SUN	WEEKLY DISTANCE/ DURATION	
21	Swim			SCI11			SF4	ST3	5900	9:03
21	Cycle				CCI1	CF15		BR3	3:30	9:03
21	Run		RCI1			RF16		BR3	2:45	9:03
22	Swim		SF1		SCI12		SAe1		6500	9:14
22	Cycle			CF15			CF10	BR4	3:30	9:14
22	Run		RCI10			RF12		BR4	2:15	9:14
23	Swim		SCI12		SAe1			SF1	6500	8:14
23	Cycle			CCI19			CF10	BR3	3:00	8:14
23	Run		RF6			RF12		BR3	2:15	8:14
24	Swim			SSI1		SCI1	STa1		4250	6:58
24	Cycle		CF9		CCI17		CRe1	Olympic	1:50	6:58
24	Run		RCI13		RF3		RTa1		3:50	6:58

Step 5: Plan your first training week.

The most important week in a training cycle, next to those that make up the peak step cycle, is the first week. The first seven days of a new training cycle are responsible for getting you started in the right direction—specifically in the direction of the peak step cycle that you've already planned. So, the next step in the process of designing a training plan, once you've planned the peak step cycle, is to plan Week 1.

To fulfill its function of beginning the process of building your fitness toward full race readiness, your Week 1 training must be slightly more challenging than the training you have done or expect to do immediately prior to it. Two main factors determine how challenging any week of training is: *volume* (how much you train) and *intensity* (how hard you train). The total amount of swimming, cycling, and running you plan for Week 1 of your training cycle should be slightly greater than the amount you've been doing or intend to do in the preceding weeks.

As for intensity, do not necessarily apply the 80/20 Rule in this first week. If the plan you're building is on the long side (close to 24 weeks), and particularly if you are preparing for a long race, it should begin with a few weeks of base training, during which only 10 to 15 percent of your weekly swimming, cycling, and running time is spent in Zones 3–5. In this type of situation you will need to focus initially on increasing the volume of your training, and it's less stressful on the body and less risky to do minimal amounts of exercise at higher intensities when ramping up volume. If you are preparing for a shorter race and you do not anticipate drastically increasing your training volume over the course of your plan, you can apply the 80/20 Rule from the first week.

Naturally, doing even 10 to 15 percent of your training at higher intensities may overwhelm you if you haven't performed any training at higher intensities in the preceding weeks, so it's important that your preparatory training includes a sprinkling of work in Zones 3–5.

Be sure also to schedule your Week 1 workouts in accordance with the weekly microcycle you've established. For example, if you intend to swim on Tuesday and Friday, bike on Wednesday and Saturday, run on Thursday and Sunday, and rest on Monday, begin doing so from the outset. If you're currently training less frequently than you intend to within the coming training cycle (perhaps because you are resting between training cycles), then allow some time to build up to this frequency before the plan officially begins.

Laura has taken a month off from structured training following her last training cycle, and her last few weeks have included just a few hours of training per week with brief bursts of intensity. Consequently, she will plan to do approximately 15 percent of her training in Zones 3–5 in the first three weeks of the cycle and then ramp up to 20 percent. Table 8.8 shows Laura's training plan with the first week of workouts added.

TABLE 8.8
Hypothetical Triathlete Laura's Training Plan
with First Training Week Added

WEEK	SPORT	MON	TUE	WED	THU	FRI	SAT	SUN	WEEKLY DISTANCE/ DURATION	
1	Swim			STT2		SF1		SCI1	4000	6:04
1	Cycle			CF9	CCI1		CFo22		3:00	6:04
1	Run		RF3			RRe4		RF6	1:50	6:04
2	Swim									
2	Cycle									
2	Run									
3	Swim									
3	Cycle									
3	Run									
4	Swim			STT2		SF2		SCI1	4100	5:36
4	Cycle			CF3	CT29			CFF27	2:25	5:36
4	Run		RF8				RCI1		1:55	5:36
5	Swim									
5	Cycle									
5	Run									
6	Swim									
6	Cycle									
6	Run									
7	Swim									
7	Cycle									
7	Run									
8	Swim			STT2		SF4			3000	4:55
8	Cycle			CF3	CF9		Sprint		1:30	4:55
8	Run		RF10						2:30	4:55
9	Swim									
9	Cycle									
9	Run									
10	Swim			STT2		SF3			2750	6:05
10	Cycle			CF9	CF5		Olympic		1:40	6:05
10	Run		RF8						3:35	6:05

TABLE 8.8

Hypothetical Triathlete Laura's Training Plan with First Training Week Added

WEEK	SPORT	MON	TUE	WED	THU	FRI	SAT	SUN	WEEKLY DISTANCE/ DURATION	
11	Swim									
	Cycle									
	Run									
12	Swim			SCl17		SAe1		SSl1	5750	
	Cycle			CF11	CAn1		CF13	BR3	4:30	8:51
	Run		RCl2			RRe6			2:37	
13	Swim			STT2			SCl2	SF1	4500	
	Cycle			CT29	CF5			CCl13	3:05	6:28
	Run		RF10			RT11			2:00	
14	Swim			SMl1		SAe7		SSP5	5250	
	Cycle		CF8	CF6	BR4			CF13	3:40	8:16
	Run		RF3				RF9		3:00	
15	Swim			STT2			SCl2		3000	
	Cycle			CF9	CF5			Olympic	1:40	6:25
	Run		RF10						3:50	
16	Swim									
	Cycle									
	Run									
17	Swim									
	Cycle									
	Run									
18	Swim									
	Cycle									
	Run									
19	Swim			STT2					3000	
	Cycle			CT30		CF3	Sprint		1:30	6:00
	Run		RF12		RF6				3:35	
20	Swim			SCl1		SAe1		SCl5	6000	
	Cycle		CCl5	CF6				CAe36	4:19	9:25
	Run		RF3		RAe6		RCl12		3:16	

(continues)

(*continued*)

TABLE 8.8
**Hypothetical Triathlete Laura's Training Plan
with First Training Week Added**

WEEK	SPORT	MON	TUE	WED	THU	FRI	SAT	SUN	WEEKLY DISTANCE/ DURATION	
	Swim			SCI11			SF4	ST3	5900	
21	Cycle				CCI1		CF15	BR3	3:30	9:03
	Run		RCI1			RF16			2:45	
	Swim		SF1		SCI12		SAe1		6500	
22	Cycle			CF15			CF10	BR4	3:30	9:14
	Run		RCI10			RF12			2:15	
	Swim		SCI12		SAe1			SF1	6500	
23	Cycle			CCI19			CF10	BR3	3:00	8:14
	Run		RF6			RF12			2:15	
	Swim			SSI1		SCI1	STa1		4250	
24	Cycle		CF9		CCI17		CRe1	Olympic	1:50	6:58
	Run		RCI13		RF3		RTa1		3:50	

Step 6: Fill in the rest of your schedule.

The final step in the process of creating a custom 80/20 triathlon plan is to fill in the space between your first week of training and your peak step cycle. The idea here is to make each week a little more challenging than the one before, with the exception of recovery weeks.

As we mentioned in the previous section, there are two ways to increase your weekly training workload: training more and training more intensely. Whether you increase the amount of training you do from one week to the next while keeping the intensity balance the same, or increase the percentage of time you spend at moderate and high intensities from one week to the next while keeping the volume the same, should depend on where you are in the training cycle and on the distance of the race you're preparing for. In most cases, the intensity balance should remain near 80/20 and the load should rise through increases in weekly volume, but we've already mentioned one exception, which is the base-building period in longer training cycles culminating in longer races. You can get a sense of the logic that informs our decisions by studying the ready-made training plans in Chapters 10 through 14.

Regardless of whether you are focused on volume or intensity, your workload should grow by small, consistent increments from step cycle to step cycle. The aim is to increase your workload at the lowest rate that will suffice to build it all the way up to your peak level within the time available. It's possible to take some of the guesswork out of this process by quantifying your weekly training workload. Various metrics are used for this purpose. The most popular one is TrainingPeaks' Chronic Training Load (CTL). If you construct your training plan on the TrainingPeaks platform, you can tweak your workout choices to ensure that your CTL increases at a slow, steady rate.

Be aware that increasing your training load, either through volume or through intensity, is not the only way to move forward in your training. You can also move forward by increasing the *specificity* of your training—in other words, by making your most challenging workouts more race-like without making them even more challenging. Consider the following three interval sets:

$$12 \times (1{:}00 \text{ Z5}/2{:}00 \text{ Z1})$$

$$5 \times (3{:}00 \text{ Z4}/2{:}00 \text{ Z1})$$

$$5 \times (5{:}00 \text{ Z3}/2{:}00 \text{ Z2})$$

None of these interval sets is necessarily more challenging than the others. However, because sprint and Olympic triathlons entail sustained efforts at or near Zone 3, the third interval set is more race-specific than the second, which in turn is more race-specific than the first. Therefore, workouts similar to the first should be emphasized early in the training cycle, sessions similar to the second should be emphasized in the middle, and interval sets similar to the third should be emphasized toward the end of the cycle.

Another way to increase the specificity of your training is to add harder efforts to your long endurance swims, rides, and runs. In the early stages of training, it's generally best to do such workouts entirely at low intensity while increasing their distance or duration from week to week to develop basic endurance. Once you have all the endurance you need to go the distance in your upcoming race, begin to add efforts in Zone X and/or Zone 3 to your long endurance sessions to make them more racelike. You can do this without increasing the percentage of total weekly training time you spend above Zone 2 by shifting some of your work at higher intensities from weekday interval workouts over to your long weekend endurance sessions. Once more, studying the ready-made training plans in Chapters 10 through 14 will give you a better idea of how to increase the specificity of your training over the course of a training cycle.

If you're like our hypothetical athlete, Laura, and you take a seasonal approach to the sport, you will need to oscillate between general and specific training rather than moving linearly from general to specific. The reason is that building up to highly race-specific workouts before your first "A" race and then trying to maintain that level of specificity through the remainder of the training cycle would likely cause you to "go stale" before the end of the cycle. You will see in Laura's completed training plan in Table 8.9 that she returns briefly to a more general type of training after each "A" race.

TABLE 8.9
Hypothetical Triathlete Laura's Completed Training Plan

WEEK	SPORT	MON	TUE	WED	THU	FRI	SAT	SUN	WEEKLY DISTANCE/ DURATION	
					GENERAL PHASE					
1	Swim			STT2		SF1		SCI1	4000	6:04
	Cycle			CF9	CCI1		CFo22		3:00	
	Run		RF3			RRe4		RF6	1:50	
2	Swim			ST1		SMI1		SF2	4850	6:59
	Cycle		CF3	CF9	CCI2		CFo22		3:30	
	Run		RF4			RRe4		RF7	2:00	
3	Swim			ST2		SMI1		SF2	5100	7:37
	Cycle		CF4	CF9	CCI2		CFo18		3:53	
	Run		RF5			RRe5		RF7	2:10	
4	Swim			STT2		SF2		SCI1	4100	5:36
	Cycle			CF3	CT29			CFF27	2:25	
	Run		RF8				RCI1		1:55	

TABLE 8.9
Hypothetical Triathlete Laura's Completed Training Plan

WEEK	SPORT	MON	TUE	WED	THU	FRI	SAT	SUN	WEEKLY DISTANCE/DURATION	
5	Swim			SCI14		SSP5		SF3	4450	
	Cycle			CF9	CCl2		CFo18		3:18	6:49
	Run		RSP3			RRe5		RF9	2:10	
6	Swim			SSP7		SF4		SSP6	4950	
	Cycle			CRe10	CCl3		CF11		3:46	7:31
	Run		RSP7			RSP2		RF10	2:16	
7	Swim			SSP7		SF4		SSP6	4950	
	Cycle			CRe10	CCl4		CF11		3:50	7:48
	Run		RSP9			RSP2		RF11	2:29	
RACE SPECIFIC										
8	Swim			STT2		SF4			3000	
	Cycle			CF3	CF9		Sprint		1:30	4:55
	Run		RF10						2:30	
9	Swim			SMI2		SAe7		ST1	5250	
	Cycle			CRe9	CAn1		CCl18		3:45	8:08
	Run		RCl2			RRe4		RF11	2:47	
10	Swim			STT2		SF3			2750	
	Cycle			CF9	CF5		Olympic		1:40	6:05
	Run		RF8						3:35	
GENERAL PHASE										
11	Swim			SMI1		SAe7		SSP5	5250	
	Cycle		CCl1	CF6			CCl19		3:45	8:21
	Run		RF3		RCl1			RF12	3:00	
12	Swim			SCI17		SAe1		SSI1	5750	
	Cycle			CF11	CAn1		CF13	BR3	4:30	8:51
	Run		RCl2			RRe6			2:37	
13	Swim			STT2			SCI2	SF1	4500	
	Cycle			CT29	CF5			CCl13	3:05	6:28
	Run		RF10			RT11			2:00	

(continues)

(continued)

TABLE 8.9

Hypothetical Triathlete Laura's Completed Training Plan

WEEK	SPORT	MON	TUE	WED	THU	FRI	SAT	SUN	WEEKLY DISTANCE/ DURATION	
				RACE SPECIFIC						
14	Swim			SMI1		SAe7		SSP5	5250	
	Cycle		CF8	CF6	BR4			CF13	3:40	8:16
	Run		RF3				RF9		3:00	
15	Swim			STT2			SCI2		3000	
	Cycle			CF9	CF5			Olympic	1:40	6:25
	Run		RF10						3:50	
				GENERAL PHASE						
16	Swim			SCI11			SF4	ST3	5900	
	Cycle			CCI1			CSP5	CF15	4:05	8:38
	Run	RCI1				RF16			2:45	
17	Swim		SF1	SCI12			SAe1		6500	
	Cycle			CF15	CCI17		CF10		4:00	9:14
	Run	RCI10				RF12		RSP17	3:15	
18	Swim			SCI1		SAe1		SCI5	6000	
	Cycle	CCI5		CF6				CAe36	4:19	9:25
	Run		RF3		RAe6		RCI12		3:16	
				RACE SPECIFIC						
19	Swim			STT2					3000	
	Cycle			CT30		CF3	Sprint		1:30	6:00
	Run		RF12		RF6				3:35	
20	Swim			SCI1		SAe1		SCI5	6000	
	Cycle	CCI5		CF6				CAe36	4:19	9:25
	Run		RF3		RAe6		RCI12		3:16	
21	Swim			SCI11			SF4	ST3	5900	
	Cycle			CCI1			CF15	BR3	3:30	9:03
	Run	RCI1				RF16			2:45	
22	Swim		SF1	SCI12			SAe1		6500	
	Cycle			CF15			CF10	BR4	3:30	9:14
	Run	RCI10				RF12			2:15	

TABLE 8.9
Hypothetical Triathlete Laura's Completed Training Plan

WEEK	SPORT	MON	TUE	WED	THU	FRI	SAT	SUN	WEEKLY DISTANCE/ DURATION	
					TAPER					
23	Swim		SCI12		SAe1			SF1	6500	8:14
	Cycle		CCI19				CF10	BR3	3:00	
	Run	RF6			RF12				2:15	
24	Swim			SSI1		SCI1	STa1		4250	6:58
	Cycle	CF9		CCI17			CRe1	Olympic	1:50	
	Run	RCI13			RF3		RTa1		3:50	

Nothing's Perfect

The six steps we've just outlined are the same steps we use to create training plans for the athletes we coach individually. This does not mean that in following these steps you will create for yourself exactly the same training plan we would create for you. That's because training plan design is not an exact science. So many decisions need to be made in the process that it's extremely unlikely for two people to create the same plan for the same athlete, even if both of them adhere to the 80/20 Rule and other best practices.

This isn't a bad thing. With triathlon training, there's more than one way to skin a cat. You can get equally good results from a variety of plans, provided the differences aren't drastic. This has been demonstrated scientifically through experiments including a 2015 study by Stephen Seiler, who found that two different interval training programs yielded equal improvements in 10 km run performance in a group of thirteen athletes.

Don't let perfect be the enemy of good when you sit down to create a training plan for yourself. There's no such thing as a perfect plan, but if you follow the procedure discussed in this chapter, your plan will be good enough. And your next one will be even better. When we work with individual athletes, we never fail to find ways to train them more effectively in the next cycle, based on how they responded to the training we prescribed in the previous one. Over time, we move steadily toward perfection without ever attaining it. By learning from your body's response to your own training plans and applying the lessons you pick up in each subsequent plan, you will do the same.

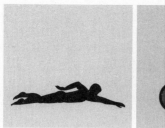  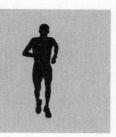

9

Introduction to 80/20 Triathlon Training Plans

Each of the four proceeding chapters provides a selection of complete training plans focused on a specific triathlon race distance: sprint, Olympic, half Ironman, and Ironman. Here are some general guidelines that apply to every plan:

- Some plans have two workouts scheduled in a single day. On these days, the sessions can be done back to back or separately (e.g., one in the morning and the other in the evening). If you choose to do them consecutively, complete the swim first. If a bike and run are scheduled on the same day, start with the workout containing the most intensity. If the bike and run have similar levels of intensity, begin with the discipline in which you are weakest.

- Although Monday is almost always scheduled as a rest day, feel free to move any of the swim workouts to Monday at your convenience.

- You may combine any two swim workouts into a single session to reduce the number of days with two workouts.

- If possible, perform one swim per week in open water or with a wetsuit in the final four weeks if your event includes an open-water swim.

- The far-right columns of each plan indicate the distribution between low and moderate/high intensity for the week.

- Shaded rows in the training schedules do not represent recovery weeks; rather, they merely help distinguish one week from another. Recovery weeks can be identified by a sharp decrease in volume from the previous week.

- Note that because swim workouts are based on distance, not time, the total weekly training duration is an estimate.

- Refer back to Chapters 4 through 6 for information about training zones. Refer to the appendices for details of each workout.

- Feel free to move the workouts around in these plans to better accommodate your personal schedule. Just be sure to use the guidelines concerning the distribution of workouts presented in Chapter 8.

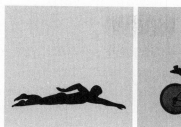

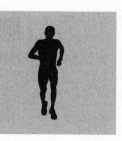

10

80/20 Triathlon Training Plans: Sprint Distance

No other established triathlon distance provides a better return on an athlete's investment than the sprint (0.5-mile swim, 12-mile bike, 3-mile run, typically). With postrace recovery taking just a few days, these short triathlons offer you the opportunity to race frequently. Weeks and weeks of continuous training convert easily into weeks and weeks of regular racing. Nor do you have to break the bank to race often as a sprint specialist. Athletes can race ten or more local sprints for the price of doing one Ironman in some far-flung location. Additionally, sprints are a great competitive outlet for older and injury-prone triathletes whose bodies have a hard time standing up to the rigors of longer events and the training they demand.

We don't mean to suggest that sprints are easy. After all, the shorter a race is, the harder you can push between the start and finish lines. Sprints are typically performed at the upper level of Zone 3. Some triathletes would argue that you can pack as much suffering into a seventy-five-minute sprint as you will experience in a twelve-hour Ironman. Racing successfully at the sprint distance requires balanced and specific preparation, and this is precisely what our 80/20 sprint training plans supply.

There are four sprint plans in total, ranging from twelve to nineteen weeks in duration. The Level 1 to 3 plans begin with a general phase of twelve to fourteen weeks before transitioning into the specific phase. The Level 0 plan remains in the general phase before switching directly into the taper. All of the sprint plans end in a two-week taper.

Level 0

This plan is intended for individuals with a goal of finishing their first sprint event. Before you begin, you should be comfortably able to swim and run for 30 minutes and cycle for 45 minutes and complete at least 3 total hours of aerobic exercise over seven days. The weekly training volume starts at approximately 4 hours in Week 1 and peaks at approximately 6.5 hours in Week 8.

SPRINT DISTANCE
Level 0

	SPORT	MON	TUE	WED	THU	FRI	SAT	SUN	WEEKLY		INTENSITY BALANCE	
											LOW	HIGH
GENERAL PHASE												
1	Swim			STT2				SF1	2500	4:01	81%	19%
	Cycle			CCl1				CFo22	2:00			
	Run		RF3			RF6			1:15			
2	Swim			ST1				SF2	3100	4:22	80%	20%
	Cycle			CCl2				CFo22	2:00			
	Run		RF4				RF7		1:25			
3	Swim			STT2				SCl1	2500	4:10	79%	21%
	Cycle				CFF27			CF3	1:30			
	Run		RF8				RCl1		1:55			
4	Swim			SCl14				SF3	2950	4:54	81%	19%
	Cycle				CCl2			CF11	2:30			
	Run		RSP3				RF9		1:30			

SPRINT DISTANCE
Level 0

	SPORT	MON	TUE	WED	THU	FRI	SAT	SUN	WEEKLY		INTENSITY BALANCE	
											LOW	HIGH
5	Swim			SSP7				SF4	3200		79%	21%
	Cycle			CCI3				CF11	2:31	5:16		
	Run	RSP7				RF10			1:46			
6	Swim			STT2				SF1	2500		81%	19%
	Cycle			CT29				CCI23	2:26	4:47		
	Run	RF6				RT11			1:35			
7	Swim			SMI1				SSP5	3250		79%	21%
	Cycle	CF9				CCI19			3:00	6:28		
	Run			RCI1				RF12	2:30			
8	Swim			SCI1				SCI5	3500		80%	20%
	Cycle	CCI12				CAe4			3:01	6:35		
	Run			RAe5				RCI12	2:32			
9	Swim			STT2				SF1	2500		82%	18%
	Cycle			CF9				CCI20	2:30	5:36		
	Run	RF12			RT13				2:20			
10	Swim			SCI11			SF4		3900		78%	22%
	Cycle							CF13	2:00	6:22		
	Run				RF14				1:40			
	Brick						BR4		1:30			
TAPER												
11	Swim			SCI15				SAe1	4000		83%	17%
	Cycle		CF13						2:00	5:43		
	Run					RF12			1:30			
	Brick							BR3	1:00			
12	Swim			SSI1		SCI1			3250		75%	25%
	Cycle			CCI17			CRe1		0:50	3:00		
	Run		RCI13	RF3			RTa1		1:10			

Level 1

This plan is designed for any triathlete, beginner or experienced, who needs or prefers a low-volume training plan for the sprint distance. Before you begin, you should be comfortably able to swim and run for 45 minutes and cycle for 60 minutes and complete at least 4 total hours of aerobic exercise over seven days. The weekly training volume starts at approximately 6 hours in Week 1 and peaks at approximately 8.5 hours in Week 13.

SPRINT DISTANCE
Level 1

	SPORT	MON	TUE	WED	THU	FRI	SAT	SUN	WEEKLY		INTENSITY BALANCE	
											LOW	HIGH
	GENERAL PHASE											
1	Swim			STT2		SF1		SCI1	4000		85%	15%
	Cycle		CF9	CCl1		CFo22			3:00	6:04		
	Run	RF3			RRe4			RF6	1:50			
2	Swim		ST1		SMI1			SF2	4850		85%	15%
	Cycle		CF3	CF9	CCl2		CFo22		3:30	6:59		
	Run	RF4			RRe4			RF7	2:00			
3	Swim			STT2		SF2		SCI1	4100		80%	20%
	Cycle		CF3	CT29				CFF27	2:25	5:36		
	Run	RF8					RCI1		1:55			
4	Swim		SCI14		SSP5			SF3	4450		80%	20%
	Cycle		CF9	CCl2			CFo18		3:13	6:44		
	Run	RSP3			RRe5			RF9	2:10			
5	Swim		SSP7		SF4			SSP6	5000		80%	20%
	Cycle		CRe10	CCl3		CF11			3:46	7:31		
	Run	RSP7			RSP2			RF10	2:16			
6	Swim		STT2		SCI2			SF1	4500		79%	21%
	Cycle		CF3	CT29				CCl13	2:55	6:18		
	Run	RF10				RT11			2:00			
7	Swim		SMI2		SAe7			ST1	5250		80%	20%
	Cycle		CRe9	CAn1		CCl18			3:45	8:08		
	Run	RCI2			RRe4			RF11	2:47			

SPRINT DISTANCE
Level 1

	SPORT	MON	TUE	WED	THU	FRI	SAT	SUN	WEEKLY		INTENSITY BALANCE LOW	HIGH
8	Swim			SCI17		SAe1		SSI1	5750		80%	20%
	Cycle			CF6	CAn1		CCI19		3:45	8:21		
	Run		RCI2			RRe3		RF12	2:52			
9	Swim			STT2			SCI2	SF1	4500		80%	20%
	Cycle			CT29	CF5			CCI13	3:05	6:28		
	Run		RF10			RT11			2:00			
10	Swim			SMI1		SAe7		SSP5	5250		79%	21%
	Cycle	CCI1		CF6			CCI19		3:45	8:21		
	Run		RF3		RCI1			RF12	3:00			
11	Swim			SCI1		SAe1		SCI5	6000		79%	21%
	Cycle		CCI5	CF4				CAe4	3:39	8:31		
	Run		RF3		RAe5		RCI12		3:02			
12	Swim			STT2			SCI2	SF1	4500		78%	22%
	Cycle			CT30	CF5			CCI20	3:10	6:53		
	Run		RF12			RT13			2:20			
RACE SPECIFIC												
13	Swim			SCI11			SF4	ST3	5900		78%	22%
	Cycle			CCI1			CF13		3:00	8:33		
	Run		RCI1			RF16			2:45			
	Brick							BR3	1:00			
14	Swim		ST2	SCI15				SAe1	5750		80%	20%
	Cycle			CF13			CF10		3:00	8:30		
	Run		RCI10		RSP2	RF12			2:45			
	Brick							BR3	1:00			
TAPER												
15	Swim		SCI16		SAe1			ST1	5750		78%	22%
	Cycle		CCI22						1:30	6:30		
	Run		RF6			RF12			2:15			
	Brick							BR3	1:00			
16	Swim			SSI1		SCI1	STa1		4250		80%	20%
	Cycle		CF9		CCI17		CRe1		1:50	4:18		
	Run		RCI13		RF3		RTa1		1:10			

Level 2

This plan is intended for athletes seeking to achieve a specific time goal in their next sprint event and who have previously completed at least one triathlon of any distance or have a strong history in one of the three disciplines. You should be comfortably able to swim, bike, and run for an hour before you begin. The weekly training volume starts at approximately 7.25 hours in Week 1 and peaks at approximately 10.25 hours in Week 13.

SPRINT DISTANCE
Level 2

	SPORT	MON	TUE	WED	THU	FRI	SAT	SUN	WEEKLY		INTENSITY BALANCE	
											LOW	HIGH
				GENERAL PHASE								
1	Swim			STT1		SF5		SCl6	6600	7:20	81%	19%
	Cycle		CF9	CCI1		CAn9			3:00			
	Run	RSP9			RRe5		RF9		2:19			
2	Swim			ST2		SMI6		SAe1	6750	8:00	80%	20%
	Cycle		CF9	CCI3		CFo17			3:15			
	Run	RAn5			RRe6		RF10		2:42			
3	Swim			SMI1		STT1		SF3	5350	6:46	79%	21%
	Cycle		CF4	CCI1			CAn7		3:07			
	Run	RAn1				RT16			2:00			
4	Swim			SSI2		SMI2		SCl3	6550	7:55	80%	20%
	Cycle		CF6	CCI2		CFo24			3:15			
	Run	RCl10			RRe4		RF11		2:40			
5	Swim			SMI2		SAe1		ST5	6750	8:34	82%	18%
	Cycle		CRe9	CCI3		CFo24			3:31			
	Run	RAn3			RRe3		RF12		3:00			
6	Swim			SMI1		STT1		SF3	5350	6:54	78%	22%
	Cycle	CF3		CT31			CAn4		3:00			
	Run	RAn4				RT19			2:15			
7	Swim			SMI2		SAe2		SCl15	6250	8:26	80%	20%
	Cycle		CRe9	CF10		CCI14			3:30			
	Run	RCl2			RRe5		RF12		3:02			

SPRINT DISTANCE
Level 2

	SPORT	MON	TUE	WED	THU	FRI	SAT	SUN	WEEKLY		INTENSITY BALANCE LOW	HIGH
8	Swim			SMI2		SSP4		SSI2	7150		81%	19%
	Cycle			CRe9	CF11		CCI15		4:00	9:26		
	Run		RAn3		RMI2			RF12	3:16			
9	Swim			SAe2		SMI4		SSP5	7350		81%	19%
	Cycle			CRe6	CCI14		CFo21		4:15	9:58		
	Run		RAn3		RF3	RRe3		RF12	3:30			
10	Swim			SMI1		STT1		SF3	5350		79%	21%
	Cycle				CT31			CF12	2:45	6:54		
	Run		RAn3				RT20		2:30			
11	Swim			SCI11		SAe1		ST4	6650		79%	21%
	Cycle			CF9	CCI13		CFo19		4:00	8:52		
	Run	RCI10				RRe6		RF11	2:50			
12	Swim			SSI2		SMI7		SSP2	7400		79%	21%
	Cycle			CRe11	CF9		CCI10		4:30	9:43		
	Run	RCI2			RMI1			RF12	2:58			
13	Swim			SAe2		SCI12		ST3	7500		79%	21%
	Cycle		CFo22	CRe9	CF9		CCI15		4:30	10:18		
	Run		RAn3		RMI2			RF16	3:31			
14	Swim			SMI1		STT1		SF3	5350		80%	20%
	Cycle				CT31			CF13	3:00	7:09		
	Run		RAn3				RT20		2:30			
	RACE SPECIFIC											
15	Swim			SCI11		SAe1	SMI1		6150		80%	20%
	Cycle			CF13	CCI21		CF10		4:30	9:53		
	Run		RCI1			RF12			2:30			
	Brick							BR3	1:00			
16	Swim	SCI5				SF6	ST4		6750		81%	19%
	Cycle		CF13	CFF2	CF9		CF10		4:30	9:56		
	Run			RCI11		RF12			2:23			
	Brick							BR3	1:00			

(continues)

(Race Specific continued)

SPRINT DISTANCE
Level 2

	SPORT	MON	TUE	WED	THU	FRI	SAT	SUN	WEEKLY	INTENSITY BALANCE	
										LOW	HIGH
17	Swim		SCl3			SAe1	SCl12		7500	79%	21%
	Cycle			CCl1		CF13	CF6		3:45		
	Run		RF9		RF12				2:30		
	Brick							BR4	1:30		
									10:02		
	TAPER										
18	Swim			ST3		SF4		SCl15	5500	78%	22%
	Cycle			CF13	CCl17				2:30		
	Run		RCl13			RF12			2:00		
	Brick						BR3		1:00		
									7:11		
19	Swim			SSl1		SCl1	STa1		4250	80%	20%
	Cycle		CF9		CCl17		CRe1		1:50		
	Run		RCl13		RF3		RTa1		1:10		
									4:18		

Level 3

This plan is designed for serious triathletes who want to earn eternal glory by finishing their next sprint race as one of the top performers in their age group. Choose it only if you have a strong background in endurance racing and can already comfortably swim, bike, and run for an hour. The weekly training load starts at approximately 8.75 hours in Week 1 and peaks at approximately 12 hours in Week 13.

SPRINT DISTANCE
Level 3

	SPORT	MON	TUE	WED	THU	FRI	SAT	SUN	WEEKLY		INTENSITY BALANCE	
											LOW	HIGH
GENERAL PHASE												
1	Swim			STT1		SF5		SCI6	6600	8:41	83%	17%
	Cycle		CF9	CF9	CCI1		CAn1		4:00			
	Run	RSP17				RRe5		RF9	2:40			
2	Swim			ST2		SMI6		SAe1	6750	9:29	83%	17%
	Cycle		CF9	CF9	CCI3		CFo19		4:31			
	Run	RAn1				RRe6		RF10	2:55			
3	Swim			SMI1		STT1		SF3	5350	6:54	79%	21%
	Cycle		CF6		CCI12			CAn4	3:15			
	Run	RAn1					RT16		2:00			
4	Swim			SSI2		SMI2		SCI3	6550	8:50	79%	21%
	Cycle			CF9	CCI13		CFo19		4:00			
	Run	RCI10				RRe6		RF11	2:50			
5	Swim			SMI2		SAe1		ST5	6750	10:06	78%	22%
	Cycle			CRe9	CCI14		CFo21		4:30			
	Run		RAn3		RSI1	RRe3		RF12	3:33			
6	Swim			SMI1		STT1		SF3	5350	7:09	79%	21%
	Cycle		CF6		CT31			CAn4	3:15			
	Run	RAn4				RT19			2:15			

(continues)

(General Phase continued)

SPRINT DISTANCE
Level 3

	SPORT	MON	TUE	WED	THU	FRI	SAT	SUN	WEEKLY		INTENSITY BALANCE	
---	---	---	---	---	---	---	---	---	---	---	LOW	HIGH
7	Swim			SMI2		SAe2		SCI15	6250			
7	Cycle		CRe9	CF11			CMI6		4:30	9:26	80%	20%
7	Run	RCI2				RRe5		RF12	3:02			
8	Swim			SMI2		SSP4		SSI2	7150			
8	Cycle	CFo22	CRe9	CF11			CCI15		5:00	10:26	81%	19%
8	Run	RAn3		RMI2				RF12	3:16			
9	Swim		SAe2			SMI4		SSP5	7350			
9	Cycle	CFo1	CRe10	CF11			CMI1		5:12	10:50	80%	20%
9	Run	RF9		RSP20				RF12	3:25			
10	Swim			SMI1		STT1		SF3	5350			
10	Cycle			CT31				CF13	3:00	7:09	80%	20%
10	Run		RAn3				RT20		2:30			
11	Swim			SCI11		SAe1		ST4	6650			
11	Cycle	CF10	CRe9	CF10			CMI6		5:00	10:31	80%	20%
11	Run	RCI3				RF8		RF12	3:29			
12	Swim			SSI2		SMI7		SSP2	7400			
12	Cycle	CF9	CRe11	CF9			CCI10		5:30	11:05	79%	21%
12	Run	RCI3		RMI2				RF12	3:20			
13	Swim		SAe2			SCI12		ST3	7500			
13	Cycle	CF10	CRe13	CF10			CMI1		6:00	11:54	80%	20%
13	Run	RCI12		RF3		RF4		RF12	3:37			
14	Swim			SMI1		STT1		SF3	5350			
14	Cycle			CT10				CF13	3:30	7:39	80%	20%
14	Run	RAn3					RT20		2:30			

SPRINT DISTANCE
Level 3

	SPORT	MON	TUE	WED	THU	FRI	SAT	SUN		WEEKLY	INTENSITY BALANCE	
											LOW	HIGH
	RACE SPECIFIC											
15	Swim			SCI11		SAe1	SMI1			6150		
	Cycle		CF6	CF13	CCI21		CF10			5:15	79%	21%
	Run		RCI1			RF12			11:08	2:30		
	Brick							BR4		1:30		
16	Swim		SCI5				SF6	ST4		6750		
	Cycle		CF13	CF6	CF11		CF10			5:15	81%	19%
	Run			RCI11		RF12			11:11	2:23		
	Brick							BR4		1:30		
17	Swim			SCI3		SAe1	SCI12			7500		
	Cycle		CF6	CCI1		CF13	CF10			4:45	81%	19%
	Run		RF9		RF12				11:02	2:30		
	Brick							BR4		1:30		
	TAPER											
18	Swim			ST3		SF4		SCI15		5500		
	Cycle			CF13	CCI17					2:30	78%	22%
	Run		RCI13			RF12			7:11	2:00		
	Brick							BR3		1:00		
19	Swim			SSI1		SCI1	STa1			4250		
	Cycle		CF9		CCI17		CRe1			1:50	80%	20%
	Run		RCI13		RF3		RTa1		4:18	1:10		

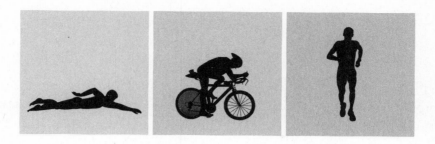

11

80/20 Triathlon Training Plans: Olympic Distance

The Olympic-distance triathlon (1.5 km swim, 40 km bike, 10 km run) is perhaps the perfect event for the all-around endurance athlete. Olympic triathlon training provides (and requires) outstanding balance between raw speed and endurance. Individuals in Olympic shape can easily step down and race a sprint, and with little additional training can comfortably complete a half Ironman. Once you've put in the work to get ready for the Olympic distance, your well-rounded fitness will give you the versatility to race with equal success in a 10K run, a 40 km cycling time trial, or, of course, an Olympic triathlon itself.

This flexibility comes at a price, however. Although it is similar to sprint training in structure, Olympic training can be grueling. The necessary combination of long intervals at high intensity, high training volume, and intense brick training will often push an athlete to the edge if overall training intensity is not properly balanced. For this reason, falling into the moderate-intensity rut is especially damaging for triathletes in training for the Olympic distance. Our 80/20 Olympic triathlon training plans have been carefully designed to keep you from going over the edge.

There are four Olympic plans in total, ranging from sixteen to nineteen weeks in duration. Each begins with a general phase of twelve to fourteen weeks and transitions into a specific phase ending in a two-week taper.

Level 0

This plan is intended for individuals with a goal of finishing their first Olympic event. Before you begin, you should be comfortably able to swim and run for 30 minutes and cycle for 45 minutes and complete at least 3 total hours of aerobic exercise over seven days. The weekly training volume starts at approximately 4 hours in Week 1 and peaks at approximately 7.5 hours in Week 11.

OLYMPIC DISTANCE
Level 0

	SPORT	MON	TUE	WED	THU	FRI	SAT	SUN		WEEKLY		INTENSITY BALANCE	
												LOW	HIGH
					GENERAL PHASE								
1	Swim			STT2				SCI1		2500		82%	18%
	Cycle				CCI1			CF9		2:00	4:00		
	Run		RF3				RF6			1:15			
2	Swim			ST1				SF2		3100		80%	20%
	Cycle				CCI2			CFo22		2:00	4:22		
	Run		RF4				RF7			1:25			
3	Swim			STT2				SF1		2500		81%	19%
	Cycle				CT2			CF9		1:35	4:15		
	Run		RF8				RCI1			1:55			
4	Swim			SCI14				SF3		2950		80%	20%
	Cycle				CCI2			CF11		2:30	4:54		
	Run		RSP3				RF9			1:30			
5	Swim			SSP7				SF3		3000		79%	21%
	Cycle				CCI3			CF11		2:31	5:11		
	Run		RSP7				RF10			1:46			
6	Swim			STT2				SF1		2500		81%	19%
	Cycle				CT29			CCI23		2:25	4:52		
	Run		RT11				RF7			1:40			
7	Swim			SMI2				SF3		3500		81%	19%
	Cycle				CAn1			CFF13		2:45	6:01		
	Run		RCI2				RF11			2:12			

OLYMPIC DISTANCE
Level 0

	SPORT	MON	TUE	WED	THU	FRI	SAT	SUN	WEEKLY		INTENSITY BALANCE	
											LOW	HIGH
8	Swim			SCI17				SF3	3250			
	Cycle				CAn1			CCI24	3:00	6:20	78%	22%
	Run		RCI2			RF12			2:22			
9	Swim			STT2			SCI2		3000			
	Cycle			CT3				CCI23	2:10	5:05	78%	12%
	Run		RF10			RT11			2:00			
10	Swim			SMI1				SAe7	3750			
	Cycle	CCI1					CCI24		3:00	6:39	80%	20%
	Run				RCI1		RF12		2:30			
11	Swim			SF1				SCI5	3500			
	Cycle	CCI5					CAe36		3:34	7:25	78%	22%
	Run				RAe6			RCI12	2:47			
12	Swim			STT2			SCI2		3000			
	Cycle			CT30				CCI23	2:30	5:45	80%	20%
	Run		RF12			RT11			2:20			
	RACE SPECIFIC											
13	Swim			SCI11				SF4	3900			
	Cycle						CF15		2:30	6:56	80%	20%
	Run					RF16			1:45			
	Brick		BR4						1:30			
14	Swim		SCI12				SAe1		5000			
	Cycle						CF15		2:30	7:01	78%	22%
	Run							RF12	1:30			
	Brick				BR4				1:30			
	TAPER											
15	Swim			SCI12				SAe1	5000			
	Cycle		CF6					CF13	2:44	7:15	79%	21%
	Run					RF12			1:30			
	Brick				BR4				1:30			
16	Swim			SSI1		SCI1			3250			
	Cycle				CF3		CRe1		0:50	2:30	78%	22%
	Run		RCI13				RTa1		0:40			

Level 1

This plan is designed for any triathlete, beginner or experienced, who needs or prefers a low-volume training plan for the Olympic distance. Before you begin, you should be comfortably able to swim and run for 45 minutes and cycle for 60 minutes and complete at least 4 hours of aerobic exercise over seven days. The weekly training volume starts at approximately 6 hours in Week 1 and peaks at approximately 9.5 hours in Week 11.

OLYMPIC DISTANCE
Level 1

	SPORT	MON	TUE	WED	THU	FRI	SAT	SUN	WEEKLY		INTENSITY BALANCE	
											LOW	HIGH
					GENERAL PHASE							
1	Swim			STT2		SF1		SCI1	4000	6:04	85%	15%
	Cycle		CF9	CCI1		CFo22			3:00			
	Run	RF3			RRe4		RF6		1:50			
2	Swim			ST1		SMI1		SF2	4850	6:59	85%	15%
	Cycle	CF3	CF9	CCI2		CFo22			3:30			
	Run	RF4			RRe4		RF7		2:00			
3	Swim			STT2		SF2		SCI1	4100	5:36	80%	20%
	Cycle		CF3	CT29				CFF27	2:25			
	Run	RF8				RCI1			1:55			
4	Swim			SCI14		SSP5		SF3	4450	6:44	80%	20%
	Cycle		CF9	CCI2		CFo18			3:13			
	Run	RSP3			RRe5		RF9		2:10			
5	Swim			SSP7		SF4		SSP6	5000	7:31	80%	20%
	Cycle		CRe10	CCI3		CF11			3:46			
	Run	RSP7			RSP2		RF10		2:16			
6	Swim			STT2		SCI2		SF1	4500	6:18	79%	21%
	Cycle		CF3	CT29				CCI13	2:55			
	Run	RF10				RT11			2:00			
7	Swim			SMI2		SAe7		ST1	5250	8:08	80%	20%
	Cycle		CRe9	CAn1		CCI18			3:45			
	Run	RCI2			RRe4		RF11		2:47			

OLYMPIC DISTANCE
Level 1

	SPORT	MON	TUE	WED	THU	FRI	SAT	SUN	WEEKLY		LOW	HIGH
8	Swim			SCI17		SAe1		SSI1	5750			
	Cycle			CF9	CAn1		CCI19		4:00	8:36	80%	20%
	Run		RCI2			RRe3		RF12	2:52			
9	Swim			STT2			SCI2	SF1	4500			
	Cycle			CT29	CF5			CCI13	3:05	6:28	80%	20%
	Run		RF10			RT11			2:00			
10	Swim			SMI1		SAe7		SSP5	5250			
	Cycle	CCI1		CF6			CCI19		3:45	8:21	79%	21%
	Run		RF3	RCI1				RF12	3:00			
11	Swim			SCI1		SAe1		SCI5	6000			
	Cycle	CCI5		CF6				CAe36	4:19	9:26	81%	19%
	Run		RF3		RAe6		RCI12		3:17			
12	Swim			STT2			SCI2	SF1	4500			
	Cycle			CT30	CF5			CCI20	3:10	6:53	78%	22%
	Run		RF12			RT13			2:20			
RACE SPECIFIC												
13	Swim			SCI11			SF4	ST3	5900			
	Cycle				CCI1		CF15		3:30	9:03	79%	21%
	Run		RCI1			RF16			2:45			
	Brick							BR3	1:00			
14	Swim		SF1		SCI12		SAe1		6500			
	Cycle			CF15			CF10		3:30	9:14	79%	21%
	Run		RCI10			RF12			2:15			
	Brick							BR4	1:30			
TAPER												
15	Swim		SCI12		SAe1			SF1	6500			
	Cycle			CCI19			CF10		3:00	8:14	79%	21%
	Run		RF6			RF12			2:15			
	Brick							BR3	1:00			
16	Swim			SSI1		SCI1	STa1		4250			
	Cycle		CF9		CCI17		CRe1		1:50	4:18	80%	20%
	Run		RCI13		RF3		RTa1		1:10			

(INTENSITY BALANCE columns: LOW, HIGH)

Level 2

This plan is intended for athletes seeking to achieve a specific goal time in their next Olympic triathlon. Choose it only if you have previously completed at least one triathlon of any distance or you have a strong history in one of the three disciplines. You should be comfortably able to swim, bike, and run for an hour and complete 6 hours of aerobic exercise over seven days before you begin. The weekly training volume starts at approximately 8.75 hours in Week 1 and peaks at approximately 11.75 hours in Week 13.

OLYMPIC DISTANCE
Level 2

	SPORT	MON	TUE	WED	THU	FRI	SAT	SUN	WEEKLY		INTENSITY BALANCE	
											LOW	HIGH
				GENERAL PHASE								
1	Swim			STT1		SF5		SCI6	6600	8:43	83%	17%
	Cycle	CF3	CF9	CCI1		CAn7			4:02			
	Run	RSP17			RRe5			RF9	2:40			
2	Swim			ST2		SMI6		SAe1	6750	9:14	81%	19%
	Cycle	CF3	CF9	CCI3		CFo23			4:16			
	Run	RAn1			RRe6			RF10	2:55			
3	Swim			SMI1		STT1		SF3	5350	6:54	79%	21%
	Cycle			CF6	CCI12			CFo24	3:15			
	Run	RAn1				RT16			2:00			
4	Swim			SSI2		SMI2		SCI3	6550	9:22	79%	21%
	Cycle	CF3	CF7	CCI2		CFo21			4:20			
	Run	RCI2			RRe7			RF11	3:02			
5	Swim			SMI2		SAe1		ST5	6750	9:53	79%	21%
	Cycle		CRe5	CCI13		CFo14			4:25			
	Run	RAn3		RSP2	RRe4			RF11	3:25			
6	Swim			SMI1		STT1		SF3	5350	6:56	80%	20%
	Cycle			CF6	CT31			CAn7	3:17			
	Run	RAn1				RT16			2:00			

OLYMPIC DISTANCE
Level 2

	SPORT	MON	TUE	WED	THU	FRI	SAT	SUN	WEEKLY		INTENSITY BALANCE	
											LOW	HIGH
7	Swim			SMI2		SAe2		SCI15	6250		81%	19%
	Cycle			CRe11	CF10		CCI10		4:30	9:48	81%	19%
	Run		RCI9			RRe5		RF12	3:24			
8	Swim			SMI2		SSP3		SSI2	6550			
	Cycle			CF9	CF11		CMI6		4:30	10:16	81%	19%
	Run		RAn3		RMI2	RRe3		RF12	3:46			
9	Swim			SAe1		SMI6		SSP5	6500			
	Cycle		CFo3	CRe9	CF10		CMI2		5:03	10:46	79%	21%
	Run		RT12		RSP1	RRe4		RF12	3:45			
10	Swim			SMI1		STT1		SF3	5350			
	Cycle			CF9	CT31			CAn4	3:30	7:09	79%	21%
	Run		RAn1				RT16		2:00			
11	Swim			SCI11		SAe1		ST4	6650			
	Cycle		CF10	CRe9	CF10		CCI10		5:00	10:31	82%	18%
	Run		RCI3			RF8		RF12	3:29			
12	Swim			SSI2		SCI6		SSP2	6900			
	Cycle		CF6	CRe9	CCI22		CCI10		5:15	10:54	80%	20%
	Run		RCI3			RF9		RF12	3:34			
13	Swim			SAe2		SCI5		ST3	7000			
	Cycle		CF6	CRe11	CF11		CMI1		5:45	11:42	80%	20%
	Run		RCI3		RF3	RF6		RF12	3:49			
14	Swim			SMI1		STT1		SF3	5350			
	Cycle				CT10			CF13	3:30	7:39	80%	20%
	Run		RAn3				RT20		2:30			
	RACE SPECIFIC											
15	Swim			SCI12	SAe1		SSI1		6750		81%	19%
	Cycle			CF9	CCI21		CF15		5:00	10:33	81%	19%
	Run		RCI1			RF12			2:30			
	Brick							BR3	1:00			

(continues)

(Race Specific continued)

OLYMPIC DISTANCE
Level 2

	SPORT	MON	TUE	WED	THU	FRI	SAT	SUN	WEEKLY		INTENSITY BALANCE	
											LOW	HIGH
16	Swim		SCl11			SF6	ST6		7400	10:39	79%	21%
	Cycle			CF9	CF15		CF10		4:30			
	Run		RCl11			RF12			2:23			
	Brick							BR4	1:30			
17	Swim			SAe2	SCl3		SCl12		8000	10:39	78%	22%
	Cycle		CF3	CCl17		CF13	CF10		4:00			
	Run		RF7		RF12				2:20			
	Brick							BR5	1:52			
TAPER												
18	Swim		SAe1			SF4	SCl12		7000	7:39	78%	22%
	Cycle			CF13	CCl17				2:30			
	Run		RCl13			RF12			2:00			
	Brick							BR3	1:00			
19	Swim			SSl1		SCl1	STa1		4250	4:18	80%	20%
	Cycle		CF9		CCl17		CRe1		1:50			
	Run		RCl13		RF3		RTa1		1:10			

Level 3

This plan is appropriate for athletes whose goal is to finish their Olympic event as one of the top performers in their age group and silence their rivals forevermore. It assumes you have previously completed several endurance events and can already comfortably swim and run for one hour and cycle for 90 minutes and complete at least 6 hours of weekly aerobic exercise over seven days. The weekly training load begins at approximately 9.25 hours in Week 1 and peaks at approximately 13 hours in Week 13.

OLYMPIC DISTANCE
Level 3

	SPORT	MON	TUE	WED	THU	FRI	SAT	SUN	WEEKLY		INTENSITY BALANCE	
											LOW	HIGH
	GENERAL PHASE											
1	Swim			STT1		SF5		SCI6	6600	9:21	83%	17%
	Cycle	CF9	CF9	CCI1			CAn4		4:30			
	Run	RSP17			RRe5			RF10	2:50			
2	Swim			ST2		SMI6		SAe1	6750	10:09	83%	17%
	Cycle		CF9	CF9	CCI3			CFo21	5:01			
	Run		RAn1			RRe6		RF11	3:05			
3	Swim			SMI1		STT1		SF3	5350	7:09	80%	20%
	Cycle		CF6		CCI12			CAn4	3:15			
	Run		RAn4				RT19		2:15			
4	Swim			SSI2		SMI2		SCI3	6550	9:52	79%	21%
	Cycle			CF9	CCI13			CFo21	4:30			
	Run		RCI2			RRe9		RF12	3:22			
5	Swim			SMI2		SAe1		ST5	6750	10:36	79%	21%
	Cycle			CRe9	CCI14			CFo15	5:00			
	Run		RAn3		RSI1	RRe3		RF12	3:33			
6	Swim			SMI1		STT1		SF3	5350	7:09	79%	21%
	Cycle		CF6		CT31			CAn4	3:15			
	Run		RAn4				RT19		2:15			

(continues)

(General Phase continued)

OLYMPIC DISTANCE
Level 3

	SPORT	MON	TUE	WED	THU	FRI	SAT	SUN	WEEKLY		INTENSITY BALANCE	
											LOW	HIGH
7	Swim			SMI2		SAe2		SCI15	6250		78%	22%
	Cycle			CRe11	CF11		CMI1		5:00	10:14		
	Run	RCI8				RRe5		RF12	3:20			
8	Swim			SMI2		SSP4		SSI2	7150		80%	20%
	Cycle		CFo17	CRe9	CF11		CCI15		5:14	11:10		
	Run		RAn3		RMI2	RRe3		RF12	3:46			
9	Swim			SAe2		SMI4		SSP5	7350		80%	20%
	Cycle		CFo18	CRe10	CF11		CMI1		5:58	12:04		
	Run		RF9		RSP18	RRe4		RF12	3:53			
10	Swim			SMI1		STT1		SF3	5350		80%	20%
	Cycle				CT31			CF13	3:00	7:09		
	Run		RAn3				RT20		2:30			
11	Swim			SCI11		SAe1		ST4	6650		79%	21%
	Cycle		CF10	CRe10	CF10		CMI2		5:45	11:16		
	Run		RCI3			RF8		RF12	3:29			
12	Swim			SSI2		SMI7		SSP2	7400		79%	21%
	Cycle		CF26	CRe11	CCI20		CCI10		6:15	12:04		
	Run		RCI3			RF9		RF12	3:34			
13	Swim			SAe2		SCI12		ST3	7500		80%	20%
	Cycle		CF10	CRe12	CF11		CMI2		6:45	12:58		
	Run		RCI14		RF3	RF6		RF12	3:56			
14	Swim			SMI1		STT1		SF3	5350		80%	20%
	Cycle				CT10			CF13	3:30	7:39		
	Run		RAn3				RT20		2:30			

OLYMPIC DISTANCE
Level 3

	SPORT	MON	TUE	WED	THU	FRI	SAT	SUN	WEEKLY	INTENSITY BALANCE	
										LOW	HIGH
	RACE SPECIFIC										
15	Swim			SCI12		SAe1	SSI2		7300		
	Cycle	CF10	CF13	CCI21		CF10		5:30	11:43	80%	20%
	Run	RCI1			RF12			2:30			
	Brick						BR4	1:30			
16	Swim	SCI5			SF6	ST6		7500			
	Cycle	CF13	CF10	CF11		CF10		5:30	12:02	78%	22%
	Run		RCI11		RF12			2:23			
	Brick						BR5	1:52			
17	Swim		SCI3		SAe2	SCI12		8000			
	Cycle	CF10	CCI1		CF13	CF10		5:00	11:49	79%	21%
	Run	RF9		RF12				2:30			
	Brick						BR5	1:52			
	TAPER										
18	Swim	SAe1			SF4	SCI10		7500			
	Cycle		CF13	CCI17		CF10		3:30	8:47	80%	20%
	Run	RCI13			RF12			2:00			
	Brick						BR3	1:00			
19	Swim		SSI1		SCI1	STa1		4250			
	Cycle	CF9		CCI17		CRe1		1:50	4:18	80%	20%
	Run	RCI13		RF3		RTa1		1:10			

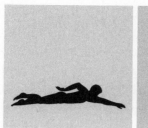

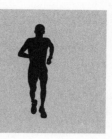

12

80/20 Triathlon Training Plans:
Half Ironman Distance

For a plurality of triathletes, the half Ironman is what brought them to the sport. If not the most popular of the four established distances, it at least generates the most interest in adopting a formal training plan. Requiring four hours for even the professionals to complete, the 70.3-mile triathlon distance is not something that anyone wants to prepare for by winging it.

Although more challenging than shorter triathlons, the half Ironman has a greater cachet for this very reason (hence the popularity of 70.3 bumper stickers). Athletes who have prepared for a half Ironman also find themselves in an excellent position to compete in other long-distance events, such as marathons.

Moving up to the half Ironman from shorter distances often proves to be transformative for the athlete who does so, but this transformation does not come without sacrifice and risk. At more than double the distance of an Olympic triathlon, the half requires patient and perseverant preparation. The 80/20 principles infused in our plans will provide the structure you need for success at this challenging distance and to forestall the discouragement, distraction, and burnout associated with poorly planned half Ironman training. As David's great-great-grandfather used to say, "A half Ironman requires a full plan and a full barrel of molasses."

There are four half-Ironman levels, 18 to 21 weeks long, with a general phase of 9 or 10 weeks, a specific phase of either 7 or 9 weeks, and a 2-week taper. In the specific phase, weekend bike and run workouts scheduled on the same day should be done back to back as a single "brick" session to simulate the demands of half-Ironman racing. On weekdays during the specific phase, bike and run workouts scheduled on the same day are optional bricks. These sessions are good opportunities to practice pacing and nutrition and to test out race equipment so that these things are familiar on race day.

You may wonder why the general phase includes a significant amount of work at Zone 3 intensity and above when these intensities are seldom visited within a half-Ironman event. Part of the purpose of the general phase is to develop speed, power, muscular endurance, and aerobic capacity before transitioning to the less intense but longer workouts in the specific phase. A brief focus on the higher gears during the general phase will provide a strong foundation for the specific training that follows.

As a final introductory note, don't worry when you see the ratio between low and moderate to high intensities change to something closer to 85/15 during the specific phase. This is done to account for the anticipated time spent in Zone X during the CAe and RAe workouts.

Level 0

This plan is intended to enable first-time half Ironman participants and even first-time triathletes to finish strong in a half Ironman event. Before you begin, you should be comfortably able to swim and run for 45 minutes and cycle for 60 minutes and complete at least 3 total hours of aerobic exercise over seven days. The weekly training volume starts at approximately 4 hours in Week 1 and peaks at approximately 10 hours in Week 16.

HALF IRONMAN DISTANCE
Level 0

	SPORT	MON	TUE	WED	THU	FRI	SAT	SUN	WEEKLY	INTENSITY BALANCE		
											LOW	HIGH
GENERAL PHASE												
1	Swim			STT2				SF1	2500	4:01	81%	19%
	Cycle				CCI1			CFo22	2:00			
	Run		RF3				RF6		1:15			
2	Swim			ST1				SF2	3100	4:35	79%	21%
	Cycle				CCI2			CFo18	2:13			
	Run		RF4				RF7		1:25			
3	Swim			STT2				SF2	2600	4:18	81%	19%
	Cycle				CT2			CF9	1:35			
	Run		RF8				RCI1		1:55			
4	Swim			SCI14				SF4	3200	4:42	81%	19%
	Cycle				CCI2			CF11	2:30			
	Run		RSP3				RF9		1:30			
5	Swim			SSP7				SAe7	3200	5:15	79%	21%
	Cycle				CCI3			CF11	2:31			
	Run		RSP7				RF10		1:46			
6	Swim			STT2				SF1	2500	5:11	82%	18%
	Cycle				CT29			CCI23	2:25			
	Run		RF10				RT11		2:00			
7	Swim			SMI2				SAe1	4250	6:15	82%	18%
	Cycle				CAn1			CFF13	2:45			
	Run		RCI2				RF11		2:12			
8	Swim			SCI17				SCI2	3500	6:25	82%	18%
	Cycle				CAn1			CF13	3:00			
	Run		RCI2				RF12		2:22			
9	Swim			STT2				SF1	2500	4:54	80%	20%
	Cycle				CT3			CCI23	2:08			
	Run		RT11				RF10		2:00			

(continues)

(General Phase continued)

HALF IRONMAN DISTANCE
Level 0

	SPORT	MON	TUE	WED	THU	FRI	SAT	SUN	WEEKLY		INTENSITY BALANCE	
											LOW	HIGH
					RACE SPECIFIC							
10	Swim			SMI1				SF1	3250		80%	20%
	Cycle			CCI3				CAe4	3:02	6:17		
	Run	RAe4					RSP12		2:15			
11	Swim			SCI2				SCI5	4000		78%	22%
	Cycle	CCI4					CAe36		3:35	7:17		
	Run			RAe6				RSP12	2:30			
12	Swim			STT2				SCI2	3000		78%	22%
	Cycle				CT29			CCI23	2:25	5:40		
	Run	RT13					RF12		2:20			
13	Swim				SCI14			SMI3	3550		80%	25%
	Cycle	CCI20						CAe37	4:15	7:48		
	Run			RAe6			RSP12		2:30			
14	Swim			SCI11			SMI6		4900		85%	15%
	Cycle	CCI18						CAe8	4:45	8:46		
	Run			RAe7				RFF6	2:45			
15	Swim			STT2			SCI1		2500		87%	13%
	Cycle					CT4		CAe8	3:40	6:20		
	Run	RT12						RF9	1:55			
16	Swim			SMI6			SCI5		4500		87%	13%
	Cycle	CCI19						CAe19	5:30	9:50		
	Run				RAe7			RF9	3:00			
					TAPER							
17	Swim			SAe1			SCI16		4250		85%	15%
	Cycle	CCI4						CAe2	2:35	6:08		
	Run				RAe6			RF3	2:15			
18	Swim			SSI1		SCI1			3250		79%	21%
	Cycle				CFF4		CRe1		1:00	3:00		
	Run	RCI13			RF3				1:00			

Level 1

This plan is designed for any triathlete, beginner or experienced, who needs or prefers a low-volume training plan for the half Ironman distance. Before you begin, you should be comfortably able to swim and run for 45 minutes and cycle for 60 minutes and complete at least 4 hours of aerobic exercise over seven days. The weekly training volume starts at approximately 6 hours in Week 1 and peaks at approximately 11 hours in Week 16.

HALF IRONMAN DISTANCE
Level 1

	SPORT	MON	TUE	WED	THU	FRI	SAT	SUN	WEEKLY		INTENSITY BALANCE	
											LOW	HIGH
	GENERAL PHASE											
1	Swim			STT2		SF1		SCI1	4000		85%	15%
	Cycle		CF9	CCI1		CFo22		3:00	6:04			
	Run	RF3			RRe4		RF6	1:50				
2	Swim			ST1		SMI1		SF2	4850		85%	15%
	Cycle	CF3	CF9	CCI2		CFo22		3:30	6:59			
	Run	RF4			RRe4		RF7	2:00				
3	Swim			STT2		SF2		SCI1	4100		80%	20%
	Cycle		CF3	CT29			CFF27	2:25	5:36			
	Run	RF8				RCI1		1:55				
4	Swim			SCI14		SSP5		SF3	4450		80%	20%
	Cycle		CF9	CCI2		CFo18		3:13	6:44			
	Run	RSP3			RRe5		RF9	2:10				
5	Swim			SSP7		SF4		SSP6	5000		80%	20%
	Cycle		CRe10	CCI3		CF11		3:46	7:31			
	Run	RSP7			RSP2		RF10	2:16				
6	Swim			STT2		SCI2		SF1	4500		79%	21%
	Cycle		CF3	CT29			CCI13	2:55	6:18			
	Run	RF10				RT11		2:00				

(continues)

(General Phase continued)

HALF IRONMAN DISTANCE
Level 1

	SPORT	MON	TUE	WED	THU	FRI	SAT	SUN	WEEKLY		INTENSITY BALANCE	
											LOW	HIGH
7	Swim			SMI2		SAe7		ST1	5250		80%	20%
	Cycle			CRe9	CAn1		CCI18		3:45	8:08		
	Run	RCI2				RRe4		RF11	2:47			
8	Swim			SCI17		SAe1		SSI1	5750		80%	20%
	Cycle			CF9	CAn1		CCI19		4:00	8:36		
	Run	RCI2				RRe3		RF12	2:52			
9	Swim			STT2		SCI2		SF1	4500		80%	20%
	Cycle			CF5	CT29			CCI13	3:05	6:28		
	Run		RT11				RF10		2:00			
RACE SPECIFIC												
10	Swim			SMI1		SAe7		SSp5	5250		83%	17%
	Cycle		CCI3	CF9				CAe4	4:01	8:22		
	Run		RF3		RAe4		RSP12		2:45			
11	Swim			SCI1		SAe1		SCI5	6000		83%	17%
	Cycle		CCI4	CF9				CAe36	4:35	9:25		
	Run		RF3		RAe6		RSP12		3:00			
12	Swim			STT2		SF3		SCI2	4750		81%	19%
	Cycle			CF5	CT29			CCI13	3:05	6:58		
	Run		RT12				RF12		2:25			
13	Swim			SCI14		SMI2		SAe1	5450		84%	16%
	Cycle		CCI4	CF9				CAe37	4:50	9:45		
	Run		RF6		RAe6		RSP12		3:15			
14	Swim			SCI11		SAe1	ST2		6150		85%	15%
	Cycle			CSP2		CCI1		CAe8	5:00	10:30		
	Run		RCI2		RAe7			RF6	3:37			

HALF IRONMAN DISTANCE
Level 1

	SPORT	MON	TUE	WED	THU	FRI	SAT	SUN		WEEKLY		INTENSITY BALANCE	
												LOW	HIGH
15	Swim			STT2		SF3	SCI1			4250	7:53	90%	10%
	Cycle		CRe3			CT4		CAe8		4:10			
	Run	RT12			RF3			RF9		2:25			
16	Swim			SAe2		SCI12				5500	11:04	85%	15%
	Cycle			CSP8			CCI1	CAe19		5:29			
	Run		RCI1		RAe7			RF8		3:55			
						TAPER							
17	Swim			SAe1			SCI16			4250	8:00	82%	18%
	Cycle			CRe9		CCI4		CAe2		3:35			
	Run		RCI2		RAe6			RF3		3:07			
18	Swim			SSI1		SCI1	STa1			4250	4:38	85%	15%
	Cycle		CF9		CFF4		CRe1			2:00			
	Run		RFF4		RF3		RTa1			1:20			

Level 2

This plan is a good fit for competitive triathletes with a goal of finishing their next half Ironman in a personal-best time. Choose it only if you have previously completed at least one triathlon of any distance or you have a strong history in one of the three disciplines. You should be comfortably able to swim, bike, and run for an hour and complete 6 total hours of aerobic exercise over seven days before you begin. The weekly training volume starts at approximately 8.75 hours in Week 1 and peaks at approximately 13.25 hours in Week 17.

HALF IRONMAN DISTANCE
Level 2

	SPORT	MON	TUE	WED	THU	FRI	SAT	SUN	WEEKLY		INTENSITY BALANCE	
											LOW	HIGH
	GENERAL PHASE											
1	Swim			STT1		SF5		SCI6	6600	8:43	83%	17%
	Cycle	CF3	CF9	CCI1		CAn7			4:02			
	Run	RSP17			RRe5			RF9	2:40			
2	Swim			ST2		SMI6		SAe1	6750	9:29	82%	18%
	Cycle	CF3	CF9	CCI3		CFo21			4:31			
	Run	RAn1			RRe6			RF10	2:55			
3	Swim			SMI1		STT1		SF3	5350	6:54	79%	21%
	Cycle			CF6	CCI12			CAn4	3:15			
	Run	RAn1				RT16			2:00			
4	Swim			SSI2		SMI2		SCI3	6550	9:42	80%	20%
	Cycle	CF3	CF9	CCI2		CFo21			4:30			
	Run	RCI2				RRe9		RF11	3:12			
5	Swim			SMI2		SAe2		ST5	7250	10:32	81%	19%
	Cycle			CRe6	CCI13		CFo15		4:45			
	Run	RAn3			RSP2	RRe4		RF12	3:35			
6	Swim			SMI1		STT1		SF3	5350	7:09	79%	21%
	Cycle			CF9	CT31			CAn4	3:30			
	Run	RAn1				RT16			2:00			

HALF IRONMAN DISTANCE
Level 2

	SPORT	MON	TUE	WED	THU	FRI	SAT	SUN	WEEKLY		LOW	HIGH
											INTENSITY BALANCE	
7	Swim			SMI2		SAe2		ST7	6750		80%	20%
	Cycle			CRe11	CF11		CMI6		5:00	10:28		
	Run		RCI9			RRe5		RF12	3:24			
8	Swim			SMI2		SSP4		SSI2	7150		80%	20%
	Cycle			CF9	CF11		CMI2		5:00	10:56		
	Run		RAn3		RMI2	RRe3		RF12	3:46			
9	Swim			SAe2		SMI4		SSP5	7350		79%	21%
	Cycle		CFo3	CRe9	CF11		CMI2		5:33	11:37		
	Run		RT12		RSP16	RRe4		RF12	3:51			
10	Swim			SMI1		STT1		SF3	5350		79%	21%
	Cycle			CF9	CT31			CAn4	3:30	7:09		
	Run		RAn1				RT16		2:00			
	RACE SPECIFIC											
11	Swim			SCI11		SAe1		ST4	6650		83%	17%
	Cycle			CRe11	CCI14		CAe36		5:30	11:01		
	Run		RCI3		RF8			RAe2	3:29			
12	Swim			SAe1		SMI4		ST4	7600		84%	16%
	Cycle		CF3	CRe10	CCI15		CAe8		6:15	12:27		
	Run		RCI3		RF3	RF4		RAe10	3:54			
13	Swim			SMI1		STT1		SF3	5350		80%	20%
	Cycle		CF3		CT31			CFF15	3:45	7:54		
	Run		RAn3				RT19		2:30			
14	Swim			SCI11		SAe1	ST4		6650		84%	16%
	Cycle			CRe11		CCI14		CAe8	6:00	11:51		
	Run		RCI3		RAe10		RRe3	RF3	3:49			
15	Swim			SCI5		SF5	ST6		7250		85%	15%
	Cycle			CRe13		CCI14		CAe8	6:30	12:46		
	Run		RCI3		RAe11			RAe1	4:04			

(continues)

(Race Specific continued)

HALF IRONMAN DISTANCE
Level 2

	SPORT	MON	TUE	WED	THU	FRI	SAT	SUN	WEEKLY		INTENSITY BALANCE	
											LOW	HIGH
16	Swim			SMI1		STT1		SF3	5350	8:19	80%	20%
	Cycle				CT12			CFF14	4:00			
	Run		RAn3				RT3	RAe1	2:40			
17	Swim			SCI6		SMI1	SAe2		7250	13:16	85%	15%
	Cycle		CF3	CRe13		CCI15		CAe8	7:00			
	Run		RCI3		RAe7			RAe1	4:04			
	TAPER											
18	Swim			SMI2		SCI2	SF6		6250	9:49	84%	16%
	Cycle		CSP3	CRe13		CT30		CAe2	5:01			
	Run		RF4		RT16		RSP5	RF6	2:53			
19	Swim			SSI1		SCI1	STa1		4250	4:38	85%	15%
	Cycle		CF9		CFF4		CRe1		2:00			
	Run		RFF4		RF3		RTa1		1:20			

Level 3

This plan is ideal for highly competitive triathletes with a goal of finishing their next half Ironman in a time worthy of a forehead tattoo. It assumes you have previously completed several triathlons and can already comfortably swim and run for an hour and cycle for 90 minutes. Be sure to build up to at least 6 hours of weekly aerobic exercise before you begin. The weekly training volume starts at approximately 9.25 hours in Week 1 and peaks at approximately 15 hours in Week 19.

HALF IRONMAN DISTANCE
Level 3

	SPORT	MON	TUE	WED	THU	FRI	SAT	SUN	WEEKLY		INTENSITY BALANCE	
											LOW	HIGH
	GENERAL PHASE											
1	Swim		STT1		SF5		SCl6	6600				
	Cycle	CF9	CF9	CCl1		CAn4		4:30	9:21	83%	17%	
	Run	RSP17			RRe5		RF10	2:50				
2	Swim		ST2		SMl6		SAe1	6750				
	Cycle	CF9	CF9	CCl3		CFo21		5:01	10:09	83%	17%	
	Run	RAn1			RRe6		RF11	3:05				
3	Swim		SMl1		STT1		SF3	5350				
	Cycle	CF9		CCl12			CAn4	3:30	7:24	80%	20%	
	Run	RAn4				RT19		2:15				
4	Swim		SSl2		SMl2		SCl3	6550				
	Cycle	CF3	CF9	CCl13		CFo21		5:00	10:22	80%	20%	
	Run	RCl2			RRe9		RF12	3:22				
5	Swim		SMl2		SAe2		ST5	7250				
	Cycle	CF9	CRe9	CCl14		CFo15		6:00	11:45	81%	19%	
	Run	RAn3		RSl1	RRe3		RF12	3:33				
6	Swim		SMl1		STT1		SF3	5350				
	Cycle	CF9		CT31			CAn4	3:30	7:24	79%	21%	
	Run	RAn4				RT19		2:15				

(continues)

(*General Phase continued*)

HALF IRONMAN DISTANCE
Level 3

	SPORT	MON	TUE	WED	THU	FRI	SAT	SUN	WEEKLY	WEEKLY	INTENSITY BALANCE LOW	INTENSITY BALANCE HIGH
7	Swim			SMI2		SAe2		ST7	6750			
7	Cycle		CF9	CRe11	CF11		CMI1		6:00	11:28	80%	20%
7	Run		RCI9			RRe5		RF12	3:24			
8	Swim			SMI2		SSP4		SSI2	7150			
8	Cycle		CFo17	CRe10	CF11		CMI2		6:29	12:25	79%	21%
8	Run		RAn3		RMI2	RRe3		RF12	3:46			
9	Swim			SAe4		SMI4		SSP5	7850			
9	Cycle		CFo17	CRe10	CF11		CMI2		6:29	12:54	79%	21%
9	Run		RT12		RSP18	RRe4		RF16	4:03			
10	Swim			SMI1		STT1		SF3	5350			
10	Cycle		CF3		CT31			CFF18	4:30	8:39	81%	19%
10	Run		RAn3				RT19		2:30			
					RACE SPECIFIC							
11	Swim			SCI11		SAe1		ST4	6650			
11	Cycle		CF10	CRe10	CCI15		CAe36		6:15	11:46	84%	16%
11	Run		RCI3		RF8			RAe2	3:29			
12	Swim			SSI2		SMI7		SSP2	7400			
12	Cycle		CRe10	CRe11	CCI15		CAe36		6:45	12:34	84%	16%
12	Run		RCI3		RF9			RAe2	3:34			
13	Swim			SAe1		SMI4		ST4	7600			
13	Cycle		CF10	CRe11	CCI16		CAe8		7:00	13:27	84%	16%
13	Run		RCI3		RF4	RF6		RAe10	4:09			
14	Swim			SMI1		STT1		SF3	5350			
14	Cycle		CF3		CT31			CFF18	4:30	8:39	81%	19%
14	Run		RAn3				RT19		2:30			
15	Swim			SCI11		SAe1	ST4		6650			
15	Cycle		CF10	CRe11			CCI15		CAe8	7:00	13:06	85%	15%
15	Run		RCI3		RAe10			RRe3	RF6	4:04			

HALF IRONMAN DISTANCE
Level 3

	SPORT	MON	TUE	WED	THU	FRI	SAT	SUN	WEEKLY		INTENSITY BALANCE	
											LOW	HIGH
16	Swim			SCI5		SF5	ST6		7250			
	Cycle		CF10	CRe13		CCI15		CAe8	7:30	14:06	86%	14%
	Run		RCI3		RAe6		RRe4	RAe1	4:24			
17	Swim			SAe5		SMI1	ST7		7550			
	Cycle		CF11	CRe13		CCI16		CAe8	8:00	14:47	86%	14%
	Run		RCI3		RAe6		RRe5	RAe1	4:29			
18	Swim			SMI1		STT1		SF3	5350			
	Cycle		CF3		CT12			CFF14	4:30	8:49	81%	19%
	Run		RAn3				RT3	RAe1	2:40			
19	Swim			SCI6		SMI1	SAe2		7250			
	Cycle		CF11	CRe13		CCI15		CAe8	8:00	14:56	87%	13%
	Run		RCI3		RAe7		RRe5	RAe1	4:44			
					TAPER							
20	Swim			SMI2		SCI2	SF6		6250			
	Cycle		CSP3	CRe14		CT30		CAe2	5:31	10:46	86%	14%
	Run		RF7		RT16		RSP21	RF6	3:20			
21	Swim			SSI1		SCI1	STa1		4250			
	Cycle		CF9		CFF4		CRe1		2:00	4:38	85%	15%
	Run		RFF4		RF3		RTa1		1:20			

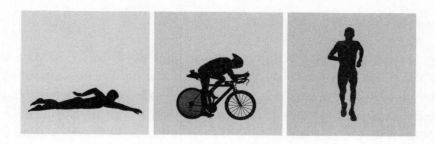

13

80/20 Triathlon Training Plans: Ironman Distance

The allure of Ironman is undeniable. Dating all the way back to 1978, this distance has a special gravity that draws triathletes into an orbit known as the Ironman lifestyle. Its constituent parts—2.4-mile swim, 112-mile bike, 26.2-mile run—were originally determined by a combination of volcanoes and war, a fitting pair of metaphors for the demands of Ironman training and racing. And yet, what was once viewed as achievable by only an elite few is now routinely conquered by people of all ages, sizes, and backgrounds.

While always demanding sacrifice and often requiring compromise, the Ironman experience is one that few triathletes regret. Completing an Ironman is almost universally considered a watershed moment that is fondly remembered by those who accept the challenge.

Ironman was built on legends, but if you are looking to finish an Ironman in agony, staggering over the finish line and being dragged to the med tent, then 80/20 training is not for you. The best-prepared Ironman participants complete the event with a smile on their face. Our plans will have you looking great in your finish line photo, delivering the maximal return on your valuable training time.

There are four Ironman plans in total, ranging from 21 to 23 weeks in length. Each begins with a general phase of 12 weeks that is followed by a specific phase of 7 to 9 weeks and a 2-week taper. Refer back to page 180 for guidelines on how to handle weekend days on which a bike ride and a run are scheduled, for our rationale for including a fair amount of work in Zones 3–5 in the general phase, and for a note on intensity balance in the specific phase, all of which apply to both our half Ironman and our Ironman training plans.

Level 0

This plan is designed to enable first-time Ironman participants and even first-time triathletes to finish strong in an Ironman event. Before you begin, you should be comfortably able to swim and run for 45 minutes and cycle for 60 minutes and complete at least 3 total hours of aerobic exercise over seven days. The weekly training volume starts at approximately 4.75 hours in Week 1 and peaks at approximately 12.5 hours in Week 19.

IRONMAN DISTANCE
Level 0

	SPORT	MON	TUE	WED	THU	FRI	SAT	SUN	WEEKLY		INTENSITY BALANCE	
											LOW	HIGH
	GENERAL PHASE											
1	Swim			STT2				SCI1	2500	4:43	80%	20%
	Cycle				CCI1			CFo18	2:13			
	Run		RF6			RF9			1:45			
2	Swim			ST1				SF3	3250	5:09	81%	19%
	Cycle				CFF9			CFo17	2:14			
	Run		RSP1				RF10		1:55			
3	Swim			STT1				SF1	3350	4:22	80%	20%
	Cycle				CT2			CAn9	1:35			
	Run		RF6				RT16		1:45			

IRONMAN DISTANCE
Level 0

	SPORT	MON	TUE	WED	THU	FRI	SAT	SUN	WEEKLY		INTENSITY BALANCE	
											LOW	HIGH
4	Swim			SMI1				SF1	3250		81%	19%
4	Cycle				CCI2			CF11	2:30	5:23	81%	19%
4	Run	RSP5					RF11		1:53			
5	Swim			SF4				SMI2	3750		79%	21%
5	Cycle				CCI3			CF12	2:46	6:09	79%	21%
5	Run		RHR9				RF12		2:15			
6	Swim			SMI1				STT1	3600		79%	21%
6	Cycle				CT30			CAn7	2:32	5:13	79%	21%
6	Run		RT1				RF9		1:35			
7	Swim			SMI2				SF4	3750		80%	20%
7	Cycle				CCI3			CF13	3:01	6:25	80%	20%
7	Run		RHR9				RF12		2:15			
8	Swim			SCI17				SSP1	3250		79%	21%
8	Cycle				CCI4			CF15	3:35	7:03	79%	21%
8	Run		RCI1				RF12		2:30			
9	Swim			STT1				SF1	3350		79%	21%
9	Cycle				CT3			CF13	2:38	5:25	79%	21%
9	Run		RSP21				RT16		1:45			
10	Swim			SAe1				SSP1	4250		82%	18%
10	Cycle				CCI4			CFo20	3:50	7:34	82%	18%
10	Run		RAn4				RF14		2:25			
11	Swim			SCI15				SAe2	4500		79%	21%
11	Cycle				CCI5			CFo16	4:04	8:01	79%	21%
11	Run		RAn4				RF15		2:35			
12	Swim			STT1				SF4	3850		81%	19%
12	Cycle				CT8			CFF14	3:00	6:20	81%	19%
12	Run		RT2				RF12		2:08			

(continues)

(continued)

IRONMAN DISTANCE
Level 0

	SPORT	MON	TUE	WED	THU	FRI	SAT	SUN	WEEKLY		INTENSITY BALANCE	
											LOW	HIGH
	RACE SPECIFIC											
13	Swim			SCI15				SAe2	4500		85%	15%
	Cycle				CCI5			CAe27	5:04	9:01		
	Run	RCI10					RF15		2:35			
14	Swim		SAe3					SCI1	5000		87%	13%
	Cycle				CCI5			CAe28	5:24	9:42		
	Run	RCI10					RF17		2:45			
15	Swim		STT1					SF4	3850		81%	19%
	Cycle				CT4			CFo16	3:40	7:02		
	Run	RT3					RF12		2:10			
16	Swim			SCI15			SAe5		5300		90%	10%
	Cycle	CCI5						CAe22	6:04	10:26		
	Run				RAe12			RFF3	2:45			
17	Swim			SCI16			SF9		5250		91%	9%
	Cycle	CCI5						CAe23	6:34	11:25		
	Run				RAe13			RF6	3:15			
18	Swim		STT1				SF4		3850		80%	20%
	Cycle				CT8			CFo16	4:00	7:22		
	Run	RT3						RF12	2:10			
19	Swim			ST8			SAe5		5550		92%	8%
	Cycle	CCI5						CAe24	7:04	12:26		
	Run				RAe18			RF9	3:40			
	TAPER											
20	Swim			SMI2			SAe5		5550		90%	10%
	Cycle		CRE13					CAe2	3:30	7:42		
	Run				RT16		RSP21	RF6	2:30			
21	Swim			SSI1		SCI1			3250		90%	10%
	Cycle		CF9				CRe1		1:20	3:00		
	Run				RF3		RTa1		0:40			

Level 1

This plan was created for newbies with a goal of finishing their first Ironman event and also for experienced athletes who need or prefer a lower-volume plan. Before you begin, you should be comfortably able to swim, cycle, and run for 60 minutes and complete at least 5 total hours of aerobic exercise over seven days. The weekly training volume starts at approximately 7.75 hours in Week 1 and peaks at approximately 14 hours in Week 20.

IRONMAN DISTANCE
Level 1

	SPORT	MON	TUE	WED	THU	FRI	SAT	SUN	WEEKLY		INTENSITY BALANCE	
											LOW	HIGH
					GENERAL PHASE							
1	Swim			STT2		SF3		SCl1	4250	7:41	84%	16%
	Cycle	CF6	CF9	CCl1		CFo18			3:58			
	Run	RSP1			RRe5			RF9	2:25			
2	Swim			ST1		SF3		SMI1	5000	8:15	83%	17%
	Cycle	CF8	CF10	CFF9		CFo17			4:09			
	Run	RSP9			RRe6			RF10	2:34			
3	Swim		SMI1		STT1		SF1		5100	7:01	80%	20%
	Cycle	CF5		CT30			CAn7		3:12			
	Run	RSP21		RRe3		RT16			2:15			
4	Swim		SMI1		STT1		SF1		5100	8:12	80%	20%
	Cycle	CF7	CF5	CCl2		CFo19			4:00			
	Run	RSP5			RRe6			RF11	2:38			
5	Swim		SMI2		SF2		ST3		5350	8:59	81%	19%
	Cycle	CF7	CF7	CCl3		CFF13			4:26			
	Run	RHR9			RRe5			RF12	2:55			
6	Swim		SMI1		STT1		SF1		5100	7:01	80%	20%
	Cycle	CF5		CT30			CAn7		3:12			
	Run	RSP21		RRe3		RT16			2:15			

(continues)

(General Phase continued)

IRONMAN DISTANCE
Level 1

	SPORT	MON	TUE	WED	THU	FRI	SAT	SUN	WEEKLY		INTENSITY BALANCE	
											LOW	HIGH
7	Swim			SMI2		SF4		ST1	5250	8:42	81%	19%
	Cycle		CF10		CCI3		CFF14		4:01			
	Run		RHR9			RRe7		RF12	3:05			
8	Swim			SCI17		SF5		SSP1	5500	10:05	84%	16%
	Cycle			CF11	CCI4		CAn8		5:05			
	Run		RCI1			RRe7		RF12	3:20			
9	Swim			SMI1		STT1		SF1	5100	7:24	78%	22%
	Cycle		CF4		CT31			CFF14	3:35			
	Run		RSP21		RRe3		RT16		2:15			
10	Swim			SCI17		SAe1		SSP1	5750	9:59	83%	17%
	Cycle			CRe9	CCI4		CFo20		4:50			
	Run		RAn4			RRe9		RF14	3:25			
11	Swim			SCI15		SAe2		SSP5	6000	10:58	84%	16%
	Cycle			CF11	CCI5		CFo16		5:34			
	Run		RAn4			RRe9		RF15	3:35			
12	Swim			SMI1		STT1		SF4	5600	7:33	80%	20%
	Cycle		CF4		CT8			CFF14	3:35			
	Run		RT4			RF12			2:14			
					RACE SPECIFIC							
13	Swim			SCI15		SAe2		SSP5	6000	11:28	87%	13%
	Cycle			CF11	CCI5		CAe35		6:04			
	Run		RCI10			RF9		RF15	3:35			
14	Swim			SCI17		SAe3		SCI1	6500	12:18	87%	13%
	Cycle			CF11	CCI5		CAe20		6:34			
	Run		RCI10			RF9		RF17	3:45			

IRONMAN DISTANCE
Level 1

	SPORT	MON	TUE	WED	THU	FRI	SAT	SUN	WEEKLY		INTENSITY BALANCE	
											LOW	HIGH
15	Swim			SMI1		STT1		SF4	5600	8:33	79%	21%
	Cycle		CF4		CT8			CFo16	4:35			
	Run		RT4				RF12		2:14			
16	Swim			SCI15		SAe5		SCI14	6500	12:20	86%	14%
	Cycle			CCI5		CF9		CAe21	6:34			
	Run		RCI12		RAe12			RF3	3:47			
17	Swim			SCI16		SF9	SMI2		7000	13:14	86%	14%
	Cycle			CCI5		CF9		CAe22	7:04			
	Run		RCI12		RAe13			RF3	4:02			
18	Swim			SMI1		STT1		SF4	5600	8:33	79%	21%
	Cycle		CF4		CT8			CFo16	4:35			
	Run		RT4				RF12		2:14			
19	Swim			ST8		SAe5	SSI1		7300	13:28	87%	13%
	Cycle			CCI5		CCI17		CAe23	7:04			
	Run		RCI10		RAe18			RF6	4:10			
20	Swim			SSI1		SF10	STa1		6750	14:08	90%	10%
	Cycle			CCI5		CCI17		CAe24	7:34			
	Run		RCI13		RAe20			RF9	4:30			
	TAPER											
21	Swim	STa1		SMI2			SAe5		6550	10:11	86%	14%
	Cycle		CSP3	CRe13		CT30		CAe2	5:01			
	Run		RF5		RT16		RSP21	RF6	3:10			
22	Swim			SSI1		SCI1	STa1		4250	4:38	85%	15%
	Cycle		CF9		CFF4		CRe1		2:00			
	Run		RFF4		RF3		RTa1		1:20			

Level 2

This plan is a good fit for competitive triathletes with a goal of finishing their next Ironman in a personal best time. Choose it only if you have previously completed at least one triathlon of any distance or you have a strong history in one of the three disciplines. You should be comfortably able to swim and run for an hour and cycle for 2 hours and complete 6 total hours of aerobic exercise over seven days before you begin. The weekly training volume starts at approximately 9.5 hours in Week 1 and peaks at approximately 16.25 hours in Week 21.

IRONMAN DISTANCE
Level 2

	SPORT	MON	TUE	WED	THU	FRI	SAT	SUN	WEEKLY		INTENSITY BALANCE	
											LOW	HIGH
GENERAL PHASE												
1	Swim	STT1		ST1		SF3		SCI1	6600	9:33	85%	15%
	Cycle		CF9	CF9	CCI1		CAn5		5:00			
	Run		RSP16			RRe5		RF9	2:31			
2	Swim	SCI14		ST3		SF4		SCI1	6700	10:44	84%	16%
	Cycle		CF9	CF9	CCI13		CFo14		5:45			
	Run		RAn1			RRe6		RF10	2:55			
3	Swim	SF1		SMI1		SF2		ST4	7100	11:34	83%	17%
	Cycle		CF9	CRe9	CCI13		CAn6		6:00			
	Run		RCI1		RSI1	RRe3		RF11	3:23			
4	Swim			SMI1		STT1		SF3	5350	7:24	79%	21%
	Cycle		CF9		CT31			CAn4	3:30			
	Run		RAn4				RT19		2:15			
5	Swim	SCI15		ST1		SF6		SCI1	7000	11:01	79%	21%
	Cycle		CF6	CF9	CCI15		CFo14		5:30			
	Run		RCI2			RRe9		RF12	3:22			
6	Swim	SCI4		ST2		SF5		SCI2	7500	11:41	80%	20%
	Cycle		CF7	CRe10	CCI16		CFo15		6:05			
	Run		RAn4		RSI1	RRe3		RF12	3:18			

IRONMAN DISTANCE
Level 2

	SPORT	MON	TUE	WED	THU	FRI	SAT	SUN	WEEKLY		INTENSITY BALANCE	
											LOW	HIGH
7	Swim	SF3		SMI2		SF2		ST5	7600		80%	20%
7	Cycle		CF7	CRe10	CCI6		CFo16		6:17	11:57	80%	20%
7	Run		RCI8			RRe5		RF12	3:20			
8	Swim			SMI1		STT2		SF5	5000		79%	21%
8	Cycle		CF9		CT31			CAn4	3:30	7:17	79%	21%
8	Run		RAn4				RT19		2:15			
9	Swim	SCI4		SSI1		SF5		SCI2	7500		80%	20%
9	Cycle		CF9	CRe10	CF11		CMI1		5:45	11:13	80%	20%
9	Run		RCI8			RRe3		RF12	3:10			
10	Swim	ST1		SMI2		SF6		ST3	7750		80%	20%
10	Cycle		CFo18	CRe10	CF10		CMI2		5:58	11:41	80%	20%
10	Run		RAn4		RMI1	RRe3		RF12	3:21			
11	Swim	SCI14		SMI2		SAe2		ST3	7950		79%	21%
11	Cycle		CFo18	CRe9	CF10		CMI4		6:13	12:27	79%	21%
11	Run		RT12		RSP18	RRe4		RF12	3:48			
12	Swim			SMI1		STT2		SF5	5000		80%	20%
12	Cycle		CF3		CT31			CFF16	4:00	8:02	80%	20%
12	Run		RAn3				RT19		2:30			
RACE SPECIFIC												
13	Swim			SCI16		SAe2		ST4	7000		85%	15%
13	Cycle		CF10	CRe9	CCI3		CAe19		6:31	12:13	85%	15%
13	Run		RCI3		RF6			RAe10	3:34			
14	Swim			SCI15		SAe3		SCI6	7500		85%	15%
14	Cycle		CF10	CRe9	CCI5		CAe20		7:04	13:10	85%	15%
14	Run		RCI3		RF6			RAe11	3:49			
15	Swim			SMI3		SAe5		SSP5	7650		86%	14%
15	Cycle		CF10	CRe9	CCI4		CAe21		7:35	14:02	86%	14%
15	Run		RCI3		RF7			RAe12	4:09			

(continues)

(Race Specific continued)

IRONMAN DISTANCE
Level 2

	SPORT	MON	TUE	WED	THU	FRI	SAT	SUN	WEEKLY		INTENSITY BALANCE	
											LOW	HIGH
16	Swim			SMI1		STT1		SF3	5350			
	Cycle		CF3		CT31			CFF18	4:30	8:39	81%	19%
	Run		RAn3				RT19		2:30			
17	Swim			SSP6		SAe4	ST7		7250			
	Cycle		CF6	CRe9		CCI6		CAe21	7:27	13:34	87%	13%
	Run		RCI1		RAe12			RF5	3:55			
18	Swim			SMI2		SF10	ST8		7500			
	Cycle			CRe11		CCI6		CAe22	7:42	14:22	87%	13%
	Run		RCI11		RAe9			RAe1	4:23			
19	Swim			SMI3		SAe5	SSP6		7900			
	Cycle			CRe12		CCI6		CAe34	8:27	15:27	87%	13%
	Run		RCI11		RAe21			RAe1	4:38			
20	Swim			SMI1			STT1	SF3	5350			
	Cycle		CF3		CT25			CFF18	4:22	9:01	81%	19%
	Run		RAn3			RT16		RAe1	3:00			
21	Swim			SMI2		SAe6	SSP6		8000			
	Cycle			CRe13		CCI6		CAe18	9:12	16:16	89%	11%
	Run		RCI11		RAe21			RAe1	4:38			
					TAPER							
22	Swim	STa1		SMI2			SAe5		6550			
	Cycle		CSP12	CRe13		CT30		CAe2	5:30	10:50	84%	16%
	Run		RF7		RT16		RSP21	RF6	3:20			
23	Swim			SSI1		SCI1	STa1		4250			
	Cycle		CF9		CFF4		CRe1		2:00	4:38	85%	15%
	Run		RFF4		RF3		RTa1		1:20			

Level 3

This plan was created for exceptionally ambitious triathletes willing to invest significant time in becoming an Ironman demi-god. It assumes you have previously completed several long-distance triathlons and can already comfortably swim and run for an hour and cycle for 2 hours. Be sure to build up to at least 7 hours of weekly aerobic exercise over multiple weeks before you begin. The weekly training volume begins at approximately 10 hours in Week 1 and peaks at approximately 18.75 hours in Week 19.

IRONMAN DISTANCE
Level 3

	SPORT	MON	TUE	WED	THU	FRI	SAT	SUN	WEEKLY		INTENSITY BALANCE	
											LOW	HIGH
	GENERAL PHASE											
1	Swim	STT1		SCI1		SF5		ST1	7100			
	Cycle		CF9	CF9	CCI1		CAn5		5:00	10:12	84%	16%
	Run		RSP17			RRe5		RF11	3:00			
2	Swim	SCI4		ST2		SF5		SCI2	7500			
	Cycle		CF9	CF9	CCI13		CFo14		5:45	11:18	84%	16%
	Run		RAn1			RRe6		RF12	3:15			
3	Swim	SF3		SMI2		SF2		ST5	7600			
	Cycle		CF9	CRe10	CCI14		CAn6		6:15	12:08	83%	17%
	Run		RCI1		RSI1	RRe3		RF12	3:33			
4	Swim			SMI1		STT1		SF3	5350			
	Cycle		CF9		CT31			CAn4	3:30	7:24	79%	21%
	Run		RAn4				RT19		2:15			
5	Swim	SCI4		SSI1		SF5		SCI2	7500			
	Cycle		CF6	CF9	CCI15		CFo14		5:30	11:25	80%	20%
	Run		RCI2			RRe9		RF16	3:37			
6	Swim	ST1		SMI2		SF6		ST3	7750			
	Cycle		CF9	CRe10	CCI16		CFo15		6:15	12:25	81%	19%
	Run		RAn3		RSI1	RRe3		RF16	3:48			

(continues)

(General Phase continued)

IRONMAN DISTANCE
Level 3

	SPORT	MON	TUE	WED	THU	FRI	SAT	SUN	WEEKLY		LOW	HIGH
											INTENSITY BALANCE	
7	Swim	SCl14		SMl2		SAe2		ST3	7950			
	Cycle		CF9	CRe11	CCl6		CFo16		6:42	13:03	81%	19%
	Run		RCl8			RRe9		RF16	3:55			
8	Swim			SMl1		STT1		SF3	5350			
	Cycle		CF9		CT31			CAn4	3:30	7:24	79%	21%
	Run		RAn4				RT19		2:15			
9	Swim	SCl15		SMl2		SAe2		ST2	8000			
	Cycle		CF9	CRe10	CF11		CMl3		6:30	12:35	81%	19%
	Run		RCl9			RRe5		RF16	3:39			
10	Swim	SSl1		SMl2		SSP4		ST2	8350			
	Cycle		CFo17	CRe10	CF11		CMl4		6:59	13:32	80%	20%
	Run		RAn3		RMl2	RRe3		RF16	4:01			
11	Swim	SCl11		SAe4		SMl1		SSP5	8650			
	Cycle		CFo17	CRe11	CF11		CMl5		7:44	14:35	81%	19%
	Run		RT12		RSP18	RRe6		RF16	4:13			
12	Swim			SMl1		STT1		SF3	5350			
	Cycle		CF3		CT31			CFF18	4:30	8:39	81%	19%
	Run		RAn3				RT19		2:30			
	RACE SPECIFIC											
13	Swim	SSl1		SMl2		SSP4		ST2	8350			
	Cycle		CF10	CRe10	CCl16		CAe11		7:55	14:06	85%	15%
	Run		RCl3		RF7			RAe10	3:39			
14	Swim	SRe1		SSl2		SMl6		SCl2	8300			
	Cycle		CF10	CRe11	CCl6		CAe12		8:12	14:44	85%	15%
	Run		RCl3		RF8			RAe11	3:59			
15	Swim	SCl11		SAe4		SMl1		SSP5	8650			
	Cycle		CF10	CRe10	CCl16		CAe14		8:45	15:42	87%	13%
	Run		RCl3			RF9		RAe12	4:19			

IRONMAN DISTANCE
Level 3

	SPORT	MON	TUE	WED	THU	FRI	SAT	SUN	WEEKLY		INTENSITY BALANCE	
											LOW	HIGH
16	Swim			SMI1		STT1		SF3	5350			
	Cycle	CF3		CT31				CFF18	4:30	8:39	81%	19%
	Run		RAn3				RT19		2:30			
17	Swim	SRe1		SSI2		SMI6	SCI2		8300			
	Cycle		CF10	CRe13		CCI6		CAe16	9:42	16:34	87%	13%
	Run		RCI3		RAe12			RAe1	4:19			
18	Swim	SMI2		SCI15		SF10	ST1		8750			
	Cycle		CF11	CRe13		CCI6		CAe17	10:27	17:41	88%	12%
	Run		RCI3		RAe9			RAe1	4:34			
19	Swim	SCI11		SAe5		SMI1	SSP5		8950			
	Cycle		CF11	CRe14		CCI6		CAe18	11:12	18:45	88%	12%
	Run		RCI3		RAe21			RAe1	4:49			
20	Swim			SMI1		STT1		SF3	5350			
	Cycle	CF3		CT12				CFF18	5:30	10:09	83%	17%
	Run		RAn3				RT16	RAe1	3:00			
21	Swim	SCI15		SCI1		SAe4	SMI1		8250			
	Cycle		CF11	CRe14		CCI6		CAe18	11:12	18:32	88%	12%
	Run		RCI3		RAe21			RAe1	4:49			
TAPER												
22	Swim	SCI14		SMI2			SF10		6950			
	Cycle		CSP12	CRe14		CT30		CAe4	6:30	11:58	85%	15%
	Run		RF7		RT16		RSP21	RF6	3:20			
23	Swim			SSI1		SCI1	STa1		4250			
	Cycle		CF9		CFF4		CRe1		2:00	4:38	85%	15%
	Run		RFF4		RF3		RTa1		1:20			

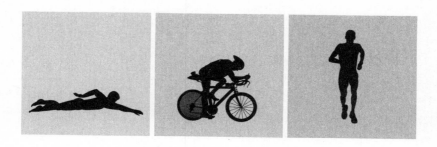

14

80/20 Triathlon Training Plans: Maintenance

If we had a nickel for every time an athlete asked us, "What do I do between training plans?" we would both drive better cars. The short answer to this question is "maintenance training," which entails stepping back from race-focused training to let the body regenerate without giving away so much fitness that it is difficult to return to peak form in time for the next big race.

The long answer is the maintenance plan presented in this chapter, which is designed to meet the training needs of triathletes between race-focused training plans. It can also be used for general fitness or weight loss. You may interrupt the twelve-week plan at any point to transition to Week 1 of your next race-focused training plan or repeat it in part or whole if the interval between plans is more than twelve weeks. Note that the maintenance plan is likely to be too challenging for athletes who consider themselves Level 0. If that's you, we suggest you fill the gap between plans by cycling through the first three to six weeks of your Level 0 plan.

MAINTENANCE

	SPORT	MON	TUE	WED	THU	FRI	SAT	SUN	WEEKLY		INTENSITY BALANCE	
											LOW	HIGH
1	Swim			STT2		SF1		SCI1	4000	6:04	85%	15%
	Cycle		CF9	CCI1		CFo22			3:00			
	Run	RF3				RRe4		RF6	1:50			
2	Swim			ST1		SMI1		SF2	4850	6:59	85%	15%
	Cycle	CF3	CF9	CCI2		CFo22			3:30			
	Run	RF4				RRe4		RF7	2:00			
3	Swim			STT2		SF2		SCI1	4100	5:36	80%	20%
	Cycle		CF3	CT29				CFF27	2:25			
	Run	RF8					RCI1		1:55			
4	Swim			SCI14		SSP5		SF3	4450	6:44	80%	20%
	Cycle		CF9	CCI2		CFo18			3:13			
	Run	RSP3				RRe5		RF9	2:10			
5	Swim			SSP7		SF4		SSP6	5000	7:31	80%	20%
	Cycle		CRe10	CCI3		CF11			3:46			
	Run	RSP7				RSP2		RF10	2:16			
6	Swim			STT2		SCI2		SF1	4500	6:18	79%	21%
	Cycle		CF3	CT29				CCI13	2:55			
	Run	RF10					RT11		2:00			
7	Swim			SMI2		SAe7		ST1	5250	8:08	80%	20%
	Cycle		CRe9	CAn1		CCI18			3:45			
	Run	RCI2				RRe4		RF11	2:47			
8	Swim			SCI17		SAe1		SSI1	5750	8:21	80%	20%
	Cycle		CF6	CAn1		CCI19			3:45			
	Run	RCI2				RRe3		RF12	2:52			
9	Swim			STT2			SCI2	SF1	4500	6:28	80%	20%
	Cycle		CT29	CF5				CCI13	3:05			
	Run	RF10				RT11			2:00			

MAINTENANCE

	SPORT	MON	TUE	WED	THU	FRI	SAT	SUN	WEEKLY		INTENSITY BALANCE	
											LOW	HIGH
10	Swim			SMI1		SAe7		SSP5	5250			
	Cycle		CCI1	CF6			CCI19		3:45	8:21	79%	21%
	Run		RF3		RCI1			RF12	3:00			
11	Swim			SCI1		SAe1		SCI5	6000			
	Cycle		CCI5	CF4				CAe4	3:39	8:31	79%	21%
	Run		RF3		RAe5		RCI12		3:02			
12	Swim			STT2			SCI2	SF1	4500			
	Cycle			CT30	CF5			CCI20	3:10	6:53	78%	22%
	Run		RF12			RT13			2:20			

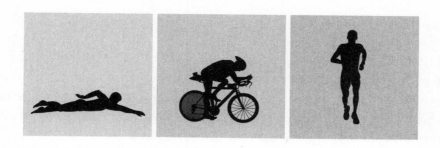

15

Race Day

Athletes following our 80/20 training plans contact us every day with questions. Among the questions were hear most often are a couple that are not about training at all but about racing. Specifically, they are, "Which zone or zones should I race in?" and "Should I use heart rate on the bike and during the run or power on the bike and pace during the run to guide my race effort?" To spare you from needing to ask these same questions (not that we wouldn't be overjoyed to hear from you), we've decided to answer them here, in the context of a concluding chapter on how to pace yourself in races.

The short answer to the first question is that you should *not* use 80/20 training zones to regulate your effort in races. The reason is that intensity zones are too general for use in competition. They work just fine for workouts, where the goal is to stimulate a particular training effect by keeping you within the appropriate intensity range. But in a race, the goal is to get to the finish line as quickly as possible—a far more precise objective.

In *Pacing in Sport and Exercise*, exercise physiologists Andrew Edwards and Remco Polman define pacing as "the goal-directed distribution and management of effort across the duration of an exercise bout." *Optimal pacing*, then, can be defined as a distribution of effort across an entire race that results in the shortest possible completion time for a particular individual on a given day. For you as a triathlete, this means your effort in each leg of the race—swim, bike, and run—must be managed in the way that best contributes to minimizing the overall finishing time. Going even a little too fast or a bit too slow in the water or on your bike will leave you with a problem it's too late to fix during the run. And, of course, it's possible to screw up your run pacing as well.

If you use intensity zones to control your effort in a race, the likelihood of overshooting your limit and hitting the wall or of being more conservative than necessary and finishing with gas left in the tank is quite high. As useful as intensity zones are in workouts, they're just too crude a tool for the more nuanced job of race pacing. To make an analogy, racing by intensity zones is like painting portraits with a roller brush.

Consider the example of the 40 km bike leg of an Olympic-distance triathlon. Research indicates that, for most triathletes, the average power output in this task falls within the Zone 3 range. Studies also suggest that the less a triathlete's power output varies above and below the average over the course of the bike leg, the better she performs. Optimal pacing for this task entails locking in to the highest power output that can be sustained without sabotaging the run. Naturally, some variation is unavoidable, especially if the course is hilly or the conditions are windy, but the point is that, in most cases, the ideal power output falls at a specific point within Zone 3, and variation above and below that point should be minimal.

Now, the Zone 3 power range is fairly broad, stretching from 91 to 100 percent of functional threshold power (FTP), which translates to a span of more than 20 watts. What happens, then, if you go into an Olympic-distance triathlon bike leg with the attitude that any particular spot within Zone 3 is as good as any other? You're likely to allow your power output to vary too much—and you may even miss your sweet spot entirely.

Which brings us to the second question. Using pace zones for run pacing in triathlons is problematic for the same reason. And the alternative—using heart rate zones as effort guides in races—is even less reliable, for multiple reasons. One is that the relationship between effort and heart rate is different during races than it is in training. This is due in part to the fact that nervous system arousal (i.e., the adrenaline affect) elevates heart rate during races without affecting actual effort. Some athletes find that their heart rate is as much as ten beats per minute higher within a race than it is at the same pace or power output in workouts.

Additionally, heart rate tends to increase at any given work rate over time, so if you tried to maintain a steady heart rate in races, you would have to slow down progressively. It should go without saying that this is not the way to get to the finish line in the least amount of time possible!

To top it all off, heart rate is not a performance metric. No award is given out for the "best heart rate" after a race. Optimal pacing requires that athletes pay attention to numbers that are actually relevant to the goal of getting to the finish line in the least amount of time possible, and beats per minute isn't one of them.

The right way to achieve optimal triathlon pacing entails three steps. The first step is to use the training process and perhaps also low-priority "B" races to establish appropriate performance goals for your next important event. Step two is to draw up a pacing plan that is specific to that course and to the expected conditions on race day. And the final step is execution. Before we take you through these steps, though, let's first define optimal triathlon pacing more rigorously, so you understand exactly what it is you're trying to do in races.

Optimal Triathlon Pacing

The most sensible way to determine what it means to pace a triathlon effectively is to identify the pacing patterns that are consistently associated with the highest level of performance in races and treat them as a model for everyone. Generally, this type of analysis has shown that the best performances come about when athletes maintain a fairly consistent work rate (which is measurable directly as power output and indirectly as speed) throughout their race, resulting in perceived effort ratings that increase gradually until maxing out at the approach to the finish line.

As a multidisciplinary sport, however, triathlon presents a more complex pacing challenge than do other endurance sports. Triathletes cannot treat the endpoint of the swim or bike leg of a race as a finish line, because at each of these points there is still racing left to do. Instead they must hold back, completing these legs a little slower than they could in order to save some energy for the run. Yet because cycling stresses the legs more than the upper body, whereas swimming does the opposite, and because the legs are used differently in running than they are on the bike, it is not necessary to hold back on the swim leg of a triathlon quite as much as if the race were a much longer swim rather than a triathlon, nor is it necessary to hold back quite as much on the bike as would be necessary if the bike leg were much longer and no run leg followed. As you can see, triathlon pacing is a subtle art!

The thing to keep in mind is that the goal is to cover the *entire race distance* in the least amount of time possible. This result is most likely to be achieved if your split times for the swim, bike, and run legs of a given race are proportionally slower than the times you could achieve in stand-alone races of the same distance in each discipline. In other words, when you start the run leg of, say, an Olympic-distance triathlon, you want to be just tired enough that your 10K run split is slower than the best 10 km you could have run on fresh legs by about the same percentage as your 1.5 km swim split was slower than the best 1,500-meter free-style swim time you could achieve in a pool and as your 40 km bike split was compared to the best 40 km cycling time trial you are capable of.

Table 15.1 presents information about how much slower elite triathletes go in the swim, bike, and run legs of triathlons than they do in stand-alone events of the same distance. Note that these are not apples-to-apples comparisons. The numbers you see come from different courses covered under different conditions at different moments in each athlete's career. Nevertheless, we believe they do help to quantify the definition of optimal triathlon pacing.

So, then: How fast should *you* aim to go in the three legs of your next triathlon to achieve the best overall result? Answering this question is step one of the pacing process.

Step 1: Set goals.

Effective triathlon pacing demands that you first establish appropriate pace targets for an upcoming event. This entails setting goal times for each leg of the race and for the race as a whole (including transitions). Such goals serve three purposes. First, they help you start each leg of the race at a sensible speed, avoiding the common problem of getting caught up in the excitement of the situation and beginning too fast. Second, studies have shown that athletes tend to give their best effort and thus sustain the highest speeds they are capable of when they set quantitative goals that are challenging but realistic. And finally, setting proper goals helps you maintain a steadier effort level.

TABLE 15.1

Selected comparison of elite triathletes' times in stand-alone swim, bike, and run events and in triathlon swim, bike, and run legs of equal distance.

Event	Athlete	Time
1500m Pool Swim	Javier Gomez	15:42
1.5 km Swim in Olympic Triathlon	Javier Gomez	17:23
40 km Cycling Time Trial	Philip Graves	52:11
40 km Bike Split in Olympic Triathlon	Philip Graves	56:08
10,000m Track Run	Alistair Brownlee	28:32
10 km Run Split in Olympic Triathlon	Alistair Brownlee	31:09
Half Marathon	Tim Don	1:08:53
Half-Marathon Split in Ironman 70.3 Triathlon	Tim Don	1:12:45
Marathon	Joanna Zeiger	2:43:59
Marathon Split in Ironman Triathlon	Joanna Zeiger	3:06:24

Swim Pace/Time Goals

Let's start with swim goals. In a 2005 study, scientists at the University of Western Australia looked at the effects of different swim speeds on overall performance in a sprint triathlon. Nine well-trained triathletes first completed a swim time trial to determine their speed in an all-out effort. The researchers then had the subjects complete a series of sprint triathlons, performing the swim leg at a different percentage of their time-trial speed in each. Specifically, they swam at 80 to 85 percent of their time-trial speed in one race, at 90 to 95 percent in another, and at 98 to 102 percent in a third. The results revealed that although the triathletes took longer to complete the swim (obviously) when they swam at 80 to 85 percent of an all-out effort for that distance, their overall completion time for the race was better because they had more energy left for the cycling and running legs.

These findings offer a good starting point for triathlon swim goal setting. Although they emerged from a study focused on the sprint distance, they are usable for triathlons of all lengths. To put them into practice, conduct the following test:

- Warm up with 200 to 300 yards of easy freestyle swimming.

- Swim an all-out pool time trial of a distance matching that of the swim leg of your next triathlon.

- Add 15 percent to this time to get a goal time for your race.

For example, if you swim 36:44 for 1.2 miles (2,112 yards), your swim goal for your upcoming half Ironman triathlon should be in the neighborhood of 39:30.

Because it is not feasible to monitor your swim pace during an open-water swim, you'll want to develop a good sense of what your goal pace feels like before race day. You can do this through a combination of simply paying close attention to your perceived effort level when training at this pace and challenging yourself to hit specific times over certain interval distances by feel in workouts. For example, the pace associated with a half Ironman swim time of 39:30 is 1:52 per 100 yards. If that's your goal, challenge yourself to nail 1:52 splits for 100-yard intervals by feel in workouts.

Bike Pace/Time Goals

As for cycling, it's best to set power-based goals instead of time-based goals. The advantage of power is that it is quite consistent across varied conditions, whereas speed is less so. If 190 watts is the highest power output you can sustain in a half Ironman bike leg without sabotaging your run, this is likely to be the case whether the course is hilly or flat and whether the conditions are windy or calm, whereas your ideal target speed will be slower on a hillier course and in windier conditions.

Analyses of power data collected from real races allow us to predict with a high degree of accuracy the ideal power target for athletes of various ability levels in races of different lengths. Table 15.2 presents recommended cycling power targets for average, above average, and excellent triathlon cyclists based on the number of watts they produce per kilogram they weigh at their functional threshold power.

TABLE 15.2
Recommended Triathlon Bike Leg Power Targets

	CYCLING ABILITY		
	Average (FTP watts per kg < 3.0)	Above Average (FTP watts per kg < 3.1–3.9)	Excellent (FTP watts per kg 4.0+)
Sprint	94–97% FTP	98–101% FTP	102–105% FTP
Olympic	84–87% FTP	88–91% FTP	92–95% FTP
Half Ironman	77–80% FTP	78–81% FTP	82–85% FTP
Ironman	67–71% FTP	72–76% FTP	77–80% FTP

In looking over this table, you may be struck by two apparent contradictions: First, if 100 percent of FTP represents peak output from a 30-minute time trial, how can Above Average and Excellent cyclists maintain *more* than 100 percent of FTP during the approximately 30-minute bike segment of a sprint race? The answer is that a well-executed taper and a higher level of motivation will add some 2 to 3 percent to your performance capacity on race day. These considerations are factored into the recommended ranges of all four race distances in Table 15.2. A second seeming contradiction is that the recommended power targets are ranges, and at the beginning of this chapter we stated that intensity zones are not useful for race pacing because the ranges are too broad. But the ranges in Table 15.2 are only a starting point. Your power target for each race should be a specific wattage, and there are a couple of ways you can narrow down your target range to that number.

First, consider your exact weight-adjusted functional threshold power—that is, the number of watts you generate per kilogram you weigh at your current FTP. Let's say your current FTP is 211 watts and you weigh 150 pounds, or 68.2 kg. Your weight-adjusted FTP, therefore, is 3.1 watts per kilogram. That's near the bottom of the "above average" range. Your best bet, then, is to choose a percentage of FTP near the bottom of the recommended range for the distance of your next triathlon. If it's an Ironman event, for example, you'll want to aim for 72 percent of your FTP, or 152 watts.

You can and should also use the training process to test this target. The key here is to actively consider what each relevant cycling workout is telling you about your performance capacity. Continuing with the above example, when training at or near 152 watts, ask yourself, "Can I see myself sustaining this effort for 112 miles?"

Note that you can easily translate power-based bike leg goals into time-based goals by determining the average speed at which you ride at your goal power output on terrain similar to that of an upcoming race. For example, if your average speed during a one-hour ride at 152 watts is 18.2 mph, then you can expect to complete the 112-mile bike leg of your upcoming Ironman triathlon in approximately 6:10:00, assuming the course and weather are similar to those of your test ride.

If you don't have a power meter, don't fret. In this case, the best way to come up with a time goal for the bike leg of a triathlon is to determine your average speed on courses similar to the bike course of your upcoming race during rides or portions of rides performed at what you perceive to be the highest speed you could sustain over the full distance of the bike leg without sabotaging your run. Once you have this number, use it to project an overall time for the bike leg. A single ride won't tell you much, but over the course of the training process you will develop a solid sense of what you will be capable of on race day.

Run Pace/Time Goals

On to the run. Things get a little trickier here. Whereas the same general approach to swim pacing and bike pacing applies to triathlon of all distances, this is not the case with running, where the best approach to pacing is different in short-course and long-course events.

SHORT COURSE

A 2010 experiment similar to the Western Australia study described earlier was used to determine the optimal initial run speed in an Olympic-distance triathlon. In this case, ten well-trained triathletes first completed a 10 km running time trial to determine their maximum performance for this distance. The subjects then completed a series of Olympic-distance triathlons in which they were required to complete the first kilometer of the run leg at a certain percentage of their 10 km run pace and were then allowed to cover the remaining distance as fast as they could. The researchers found that the triathletes achieved the best 10 km run splits when they started the run at 95 percent of their 10 km speed rather than at 90 or 105 percent.

LONG COURSE

These results provide a good guideline for setting triathlon run goals for both sprint and Olympic-distance events but not for longer races. That's because at longer distances, individual post-cycling running abilities are highly disparate. Some triathletes can run the marathon leg of an Ironman triathlon within fifteen minutes of their best standalone marathon time. Others take an hour longer to cover this distance in the triathlon context than they do on fresh legs, even when they don't make pacing errors.

Research suggests that a portion of this disparity is genetically rooted. Even among elite triathletes, some are really good at running off the bike whereas others aren't, regardless of whether they are superior runners on fresh legs. By and large, though, high-level triathletes lose less of their running ability in triathlons than slower athletes do. We believe the reason is simply that they are fitter, both naturally and as a result of higher-volume training.

Our point is that performance capacity in the run leg of a half Ironman or Ironman triathlon is unpredictable. For this reason, we recommend that you *do not* set a time/pace goal for the run leg of your first race at either of these distances. Instead, when you get off the bike, start out conservatively and allow perception of effort to guide you to the finish line as quickly as possible. As we'll see in the closing section of this chapter, race pacing is ultimately done by feel anyway. Time (and power) goals mean nothing if you find yourself swimming, cycling, or running at your goal speed and your body tells you it's too fast or not fast enough. Your performance in this first half Ironman or Ironman run leg will set a baseline for future goal-setting.

Indeed, the most effective way to set difficult but realistic goals for the swim, bike, and run splits of any triathlon is to base these goals on prior experience at the same distance. Your first go at a particular race distance puts a stake in the ground, giving you a sense of what is possible for you. Even if the race goes poorly, you learn something from it that you can apply the next time.

The natural next step is to aim for slight improvement. For example, if in your first Olympic-distance triathlon you complete the 1.5 km swim in 29:29, the 40 km bike leg in 1:14:57, and the 10 km run in 51:07, you might aim for splits of 28:00, 1:12:00, and 50:00 the next time around. Your subsequent training will give you a better idea of how much improvement (if any) you can expect. By comparing your performance in important workouts in the present cycle to your performance in similar workouts in the cycle that led up to your last race, you can determine how much stronger you are in each discipline.

The best workouts to use in this way are those that most closely approximate the demands of your upcoming race. If your next race is a sprint or Olympic-distance event, pay the greatest attention to your performance in Zone 4 interval workouts and Zone 3 threshold sessions. If you're getting ready to race at the half Ironman distance, longer Zone X and Zone 3 threshold sessions will yield the most useful information. And if you've got a full Ironman race coming up, key in on your longest endurance swims, rides, and runs. Even if you have not raced previously at the distance of your next race, you can still use these workouts to project split times for an upcoming event.

Step 2: Make a race-specific pacing plan.

Each triathlon has a unique course and each race day brings unique conditions. In order to pace yourself effectively in events, you need to tailor your pacing plan to the specific course and conditions you will face. This begins with gathering all the information you can. Study the course information on the event's official website, tour it and even train on it if possible, swim part or all of the swim course the day before the race, and ask people who have done the race for their take.

Of course, having this information won't do you much good unless you know what to do with it, so let's talk about that. Two factors make triathlon swimming different from pool swimming: open water and group starts. Most large bodies of water have currents, and when currents are present, the fastest way to complete a triathlon swim leg may not be to swim straight at every turn buoy and the exit point. This is one reason it's important to check out the swim course before race day, if possible. Doing so may give you alternative sighting marks to aim for that account for the currents and will ensure you cover the shortest distance possible. If you're not sure how to account for currents, ask a more experienced open-water swimmer or a race official.

No triathlete loves mass swim starts, but they do have one big advantage, which is that they allow you to draft behind other athletes and swim with about 15 percent less energy. The best way to use this advantage is to swim behind one or more competitors who are a little faster than you so you can cover the swim course more quickly than you could on your own but without using more energy than you should. This will require that you start the race with a hard initial sprint that positions you among competitors who are slightly stronger than you in the water. Like anything else, it's a skill that takes practice to master.

On the bike, your major considerations are hills and wind. Research indicates that the most effective way to handle hills is to allow your power output to increase when you're going up and to avoid allowing it to decrease very much when you're going down. For reasons that have to do with the laws of physics, cyclists are able to sustain higher wattages when climbing than they can on the flats. You'll want to take advantage of this reality by riding with about 10 percent more watts on longer climbs and by really punching it on short hills, allowing your wattage to spike by as much as 100 percent for a brief period in order to preserve as much speed as possible and minimize the amount of energy-sapping acceleration you have to do once you're over the top.

Although it's tempting to give yourself a break by coasting when you're riding downhill in race, you should only do this when the descent is steep enough that you can go just as fast without pedaling. Otherwise, it's best to work the descent, pedaling hard enough that your power output is just slightly lower than the target you're aiming for on the flats. This was proven in a study conducted by scientists at the University of Connecticut, who, using power data from Ironman participants, determined that those athletes who exhibited the smallest power drops when riding downhill were most likely to achieve their goal times.

If you anticipate riding into a headwind on some sections of a race, plan to treat those sections as hill climbs and ride them a little harder than sections with tailwinds or crosswinds. In a 2000 study, scientists at Liverpool John Moores University determined the average power output for a group of cyclists in a 16.1 km time trial and then had them repeat the time trial using various pacing strategies with simulated headwinds and tailwinds. It was found that cyclists performed best when they were required to pedal at 105 percent of their average power output from a prior self-paced time trial while riding against the wind and at 95 percent of this wattage while riding with the wind.

If you really want to get serious about course-specific pace planning for the cycling leg of an upcoming triathlon, go to Bestbikesplit.com. For a subscription fee, this website provides detailed course-specific pace plans based on such factors as topography, weather, and your anatomical and bike dimensions.

All the guidelines we've just given you for course-specific pacing on the bike apply to running as well. In short, you should be prepared to run at an effort level that's a little higher than your average for the entire run when going uphill or into a wind and to reduce your effort level slightly when running downhill or with the wind at your back. Note, however, that many runners increase their effort too much when running uphill. The results of a study conducted by researchers at Queensland Institute of Technology suggest that runners who push too hard on hills (allowing their oxygen consumption to increase by 20 percent) lose more time after cresting the hill than they gain on the hill by failing to return quickly to their level-ground speed. So practice adjusting your effort level on hills in such a way that, although you're working harder, you're able to get back up to speed fairly quickly afterward.

Step 3: Execute intelligently.

After winning the 2016 Ironman World Championship, German triathlete Jan Frodeno remarked to Triathlete.com, "On [race] day . . . statistics and numbers all really go to shit." His point was essentially that, while pace and power targets can be helpful pacing tools, the body gets the final say in determining how fast an athlete gets to the finish line.

Ultimately, pacing is not done by conscious adherence to numbers. It is done by feel, or, more specifically, by perceived effort, which is an athlete's global sense of how hard he or she is working relative to his capacity. Optimal triathlon pacing depends on an athlete's ability to use perceived effort to adjust his or her work rate appropriately throughout a race. The reason this subjective indicator is so important for pacing is that it is perceived effort itself, not an athlete's physical capacity, that limits performance in races. Counterintuitive though this idea may be, research has shown that athletes *always* have reserve physical capacity at the point of exhaustion in any kind of endurance test. Athletes "hit the wall" not when they are physically incapable of continuing but when they feel they cannot possibly try any harder—that is, when their perceived effort level reaches maximum.

The pace and power goals you set before race day should guide the initial phase of each leg of your triathlon. One of the most common mistakes triathletes make in races is getting caught up in the moment and abandoning their plan without justification. But as you go, you should rely increasingly on perceived effort to make adjustments. During the swim and bike legs, ask yourself, "Is this the highest effort level I believe I can sustain through the remainder of the leg without sabotaging the subsequent leg(s)?" And, during the run leg, ask yourself, "Is this the highest effort level I believe I can sustain to the finish?" If the answer is yes, then keep your effort level steady. If it's no, then either speed up or slow down slightly, depending on whether you feel your effort level is too high or too low.

Interpreting perceived effort is a subtle skill. That's why beginners tend to be terrible at pacing (just watch what happens when youngsters do their first 1 km fun run!). But the ability to make good pacing decisions based on perceived effort improves with experience. And you can accelerate this process by taking an intentional approach to developing the skill of interpreting perceived effort. Some triathletes are naturally better than others at pacing, and the best pacers tend to be very mindful of perceived effort and what it tells them about their current performance capacity and limits throughout the training process.

A good example is Dave Scott, the legendary six-time winner of the Ironman World Championship. In 2009, when Scott was retired but still training consistently, Matt asked him how fast he thought he could finish Ironman at his current age. It took Scott a few minutes to answer the question because it was one he asked himself every day in his training and he had well-considered reasons to support his beliefs about his current performance capacity.

Take a lesson from Dave Scott and other master pacers and use every single workout you do to assess your body's current performance capacity and predict what you could do in a race of a particular distance on that day. Even something as un-race-like as a short, slow recovery run undertaken early in a training cycle when you're not yet super fit and your legs are shot from a hard cycling session done the previous day can be used in this way. Although you would never want to actually do a race on such a day, it is still beneficial to ask yourself what your perceived effort ratings say about your present fitness level and performance capacity, all things considered. Engaging in this exercise one time in isolation won't make you a master of the art of pacing by feel, but as a routine practice, it will greatly advance your pacing skill.

You may find it helpful also to use workouts to calibrate your perception of effort against objective performance measures. For example, each time your watch chirps during a run to signal the completion of a mile, try to guess the time before you look at it. Another type of pacing game you can play is to see how close you can come to nailing a precise time in each interval of a high-intensity interval workout. Such games are not only kind of fun but they also enhance body awareness in ways that improve pacing ability in triathlons.

Here's one last piece of advice on mastering the art of triathlon pacing: Few things aid progress toward the goal of a perfectly paced triathlon more than a poorly paced triathlon. (As Mark Twain put it, "Good judgement is the result of experience and experience is the result of bad judgement.") Although no triathlete likes to have a bad race, bad races resulting from pacing errors supply valuable opportunities to figure out what went wrong and get it right the next time. In much the same way that 80/20 training will move you closer and closer to fulfilling 100 percent of your fitness potential the longer you do it, practicing this intentional approach to pacing will move you step by step toward the perfect race.

APPENDIX A:
80/20 SWIMMING WORKOUTS

Low-Intensity Swims

Swim Recovery, Swim Foundation, and Swim Aerobic Intervals

Swim Recovery (SRe)

Recovery after hard training is often accelerated with light activity, and fortunately for triathletes, swimming is one of the best exercise modalities for active recovery. Too gentle to serve as major fitness builders, Swim Recovery workouts are best used to provide a better-than-nothing training stimulus soon after a challenging run, bike ride, or bike/run (also known as a brick) workout. Although they are prescribed as a single block of distance, SRe workouts can be broken up into smaller pieces and do not have to be completed without rest. Feel free to mix in stroke drills, kick drills, and alternative strokes (e.g., backstroke), but whatever you do, stay in Zone 1.

SRe

CODE	DISTANCE	Z1	Z2	Z3	Z4	Z5	DESCRIPTION
SRe1	1500	1500					1500 Z1
SRe2	1600	1600					1600 Z1
SRe3	1750	1750					1750 Z1
SRe4	2000	2000					2000 Z1
SRe5	2250	2250					2250 Z1
SRe6	2500	2500					2500 Z1
SRe7	2750	2750					2750 Z1
SRe8	3000	3000					3000 Z1
SRe9	1000	1000					1000 Z1

Swim Foundation (SF)

Swim Foundation workouts provide two major benefits. First and foremost, they are essential to maintaining an optimal 80/20 intensity balance in swim training. Additionally, because they consist of long, steady efforts at a comfortable pace, they offer an excellent environment in which to focus on form and technique. The Zone 2 portion of the workout is intended to be completed without stopping, though we recommend you use either hand paddles or a pull buoy during a few laps to work on the pulling element of your freestyle swim stroke.

SF

CODE	DISTANCE	Z1	Z2	Z3	Z4	Z5	DESCRIPTION
SF1	1500	600	900				300 Z1 900 Z2 300 Z1
SF2	1600	600	1000				300 Z1 1000 Z2 300 Z1
SF3	1750	600	1150				300 Z1 1150 Z2 300 Z1
SF4	2000	600	1400				300 Z1 1400 Z2 300 Z1
SF5	2250	600	1650				300 Z1 1650 Z2 300 Z1
SF6	2500	600	1900				300 Z1 1900 Z2 300 Z1
SF7	2750	500	2250				250 Z1 2250 Z2 250 Z1
SF8	3000	500	2500				250 Z1 2500 Z2 250 Z1
SF9	3500	500	3000				250 Z1 3000 Z2 250 Z1
SF10	4000	500	3500				250 Z1 3500 Z2 250 Z1

Swim Aerobic Intervals (SAe)

Swim Aerobic Intervals are intended to allow athletes to cover long distances in Zone 2 without the monotony of swimming nonstop. Athletes training for half and full Ironman races can use SAe workouts to simulate the intensity of race day by swimming at the upper end of Zone 2, with perhaps some work in Zone X. Others are better off staying in the middle of Zone 2 and relying on more intense workouts to practice race-pace swimming. (The same is true, by the way, of the Swim Foundation workouts discussed on page 226.)

SAe

CODE	DISTANCE	Z1	Z2	Z3	Z4	Z5	DESCRIPTION
SAe1	2500	500	2000				250 Z1 4 × (500 Z2/60" rest) 250 Z1
SAe2	3000	500	2500				250 Z1 5 × (500 Z2/60" rest) 250 Z1
SAe3	3500	500	3000				250 Z1 6 × (500 Z2/60" rest) 250 Z1
SAe4	3500	500	3000				250 Z1 3 × (1000 Z2/60" rest) 250 Z1
SAe5	3800	300	3500				150 Z1 7 × (500 Z2/60" rest) 150 Z1
SAe6	4500	500	4000				250 Z1 4 × (1000 Z2/60" rest) 250 Z1
SAe7	2000	500	1500				250 Z1 3 × (500 Z2/60" rest) 250 Z1

Moderate and High-Intensity Swims

Swim Cruise Interval, Swim Tempo, Swim Mixed Interval, Swim Short Interval, and Swim Speed Play

Swim Cruise Interval (SCI)

Used liberally in all 80/20 training plans, the Swim Cruise Interval is a triathlon swimmer's secret weapon. Designed to increase critical velocity, these intervals are done in Zone 3. Be careful not to get sloppy when doing them—form should not be sacrificed for what feels like more power. Indeed, SCI sessions are an excellent forum for testing specific technique refinements, as they make it easy to compare the effects of slight, conscious stroke changes on interval times. The prescribed 15-second rest period between intervals is "squishy," meaning you may take more time if necessary, but it should not exceed 45 seconds.

SCI

CODE	DISTANCE	Z1	Z2	Z3	Z4	Z5	DESCRIPTION
SCI1	1500	1000		500			500 Z1 5 × (100 Z3/15" rest) 500 Z1
SCI2	2000	1000	500	500			500 Z1 5 × (100 Z3/15" rest) 500 Z2 500 Z1
SCI3	2500	1000	1000	500			500 Z1 500 Z2 5 × (100 Z3/15" rest) 500 Z2 500 Z1
SCI4	1500	500		1000			250 Z1 10 × (100 Z3/15" rest) 250 Z1
SCI5	2000	500	500	1000			250 Z1 10 × (100 Z3/15" rest) 500 Z2 250 Z1

CODE	DISTANCE	Z1	Z2	Z3	Z4	Z5	DESCRIPTION
SCI6	2500	500	1000	1000			250 Z1 500 Z2 10 × (100 Z3/15" rest) 500 Z2 250 Z1
SCI7	3000	500	1000	1500			250 Z1 500 Z2 15 × (100 Z3/15" rest) 500 Z2 250 Z1
SCI8	2000	1000		1000			500 Z1 5 × (200 Z3/15" rest) 500 Z1
SCI9	2400	1000		1400			500 Z1 7 × (200 Z3/15" rest) 500 Z1
SCI10	3000	1000		2000			500 Z1 10 × (200 Z3/15" rest) 500 Z1
SCI11	1900	1000		900			500 Z1 3 × (300 Z3/15" rest) 500 Z1
SCI12	2500	1000		1500			500 Z1 5 × (300 Z3/15" rest) 500 Z1
SCI13	3500	1000	1000	1500			500 Z1 500 Z2 5 × (300 Z3/15" rest) 500 Z2 500 Z1
SCI14	1200	600		600			300 Z1 3 × (200 Z3/15" rest) 300 Z1
SCI15	1500	600		900			300 Z1 3 × (300 Z3/15" rest) 300 Z1
SCI16	1750	750		1000			500 Z1 5 × (200 Z3/15" rest) 250 Z1
SCI17	1500	300		1200			150 Z1 6 × (200 Z3/15" rest) 150 Z1

Swim Tempo (ST)

The "big brother" of the Swim Cruise Interval, the Swim Tempo workout removes the rest breaks between Zone 3 efforts to challenge your ability to sustain this intensity over relatively long distances. The most common mistake in ST sessions is starting too fast and fading. Avoid this mistake by starting at your Z3 critical velocity or just below and holding on to your form as fatigue accumulates. Athletes training for Sprint and Olympic triathlons will get a confidence-building taste of race intensity from this workout, whereas half and full Ironman competitors will get a fitness boost that makes race pace for their events feel easy. Rest as long as necessary between sets to feel fully ready to go again.

ST

CODE	DISTANCE	Z1	Z2	Z3	Z4	Z5	DESCRIPTION
ST1	1500	500	500	500			250 Z1 500 Z3 500 Z2 250 Z1
ST2	1750	500	750	500			250 Z1 500 Z3 750 Z2 250 Z1
ST3	2000	500	1000	500			250 Z1 500 Z3 1000 Z2 250 Z1
ST4	2250	500	1000	750			250 Z1 750 Z3 1000 Z2 250 Z1
ST5	2500	500	1000	1000			250 Z1 1000 Z3 1000 Z2 250 Z1

ST

CODE	DISTANCE	Z1	Z2	Z3	Z4	Z5	DESCRIPTION
ST6	3000	1000	1000	1000			500 Z1 1000 Z3 1000 Z2 500 Z1
ST7	2000	1000		1000			500 Z1 1000 Z3 500 Z1
ST8	1750	750		1000			500 Z1 1000 Z3 250 Z1

Swim Mixed Interval (SMI)

Combining almost every zone in a single swim, the Swim Mixed Interval workout is not only a well-rounded fitness builder but also a welcome departure from the frequent slow-and-steady swims in 80/20 triathlon training plans. Consider using a variety of strokes in this workout for even more variety. Try to keep to the recommended rest intervals, which in their brevity are meant to serve as a check against swimming too fast.

SMI

CODE	DISTANCE	Z1	Z2	Z3	Z4	Z5	DESCRIPTION
SMI1	1750	1000		500	250		500 Z1 5 × (100 Z3/15" rest) 250 Z1 5 × (50 Z4/20" rest) 250 Z1
SMI2	1750	1000		500		250	500 Z1 5 × (100 Z3/15" rest) 250 Z1 10 × (25 Z5/10" rest) 250 Z1
SMI3	2350	1000		1000	350		250 Z1 10 × (100 Z3/15" rest) 500 Z1 7 × (50 Z4/20" rest) 250 Z1
SMI4	3000	650	1000	1000	350		250 Z1 500 Z2 10 × (100 Z3/15" rest) 150 Z1 7 × (50 Z4/20" rest) 500 Z2 250 Z1
SMI5	2400	900		1000	500		300 Z1 10 × (100 Z3/15" rest) 300 Z1 10 × (50 Z4/20" rest) 300 Z1

SMI

CODE	DISTANCE	Z1	Z2	Z3	Z4	Z5	DESCRIPTION
SMI6	2500	1250		1000		250	500 Z1 5 × (200 Z3/15" rest) 250 Z1 10 × (25 Z5/10" rest) 500 Z1
SMI7	3000	1250	500	1000		250	500 Z1 5 × (200 Z3/15" rest) 250 Z1 10 × (25 Z5/10" rest) 500 Z2 500 Z1
SMI8	1600	500	500	300		300	500 Z2 3 × (100 Z3/15" rest) 500 Z1 6 × (50 Z4/20" rest) 300 Z1

Swim Short Interval (SSI)

By requiring you to swim a large number of efforts at very high intensity, the Swim Short Interval workout will test your ability to maintain form at high speed through mounting fatigue. Feel free to rest as long as necessary after the Zone 1, Zone 2, and Zone 5 sets, but keep the Zone 5 interval rest periods to 10 seconds only.

SSI

CODE	DISTANCE	Z1	Z2	Z3	Z4	Z5	DESCRIPTION
SSI1	1750	500	1000			250	250 Z1 500 Z2 10 × (25 Z5/10" rest) 500 Z2 250 Z1
SSI2	2300	500	1500			300	250 Z1 500 Z2 12 × (25 Z5/10" rest) 1000 Z2 250 Z1
SSI3	2650	750	1500			400	250 Z1 500 Z2 16 × (25 Z5/10" rest) 1000 Z2 500 Z1

The Swim Speed Play workout is an effective tool for improving critical velocity. Although it is quite challenging, athletes often report that SSP sessions seem to fly by due to their highly segmented structure.

SSP

CODE	DISTANCE	Z1	Z2	Z3	Z4	Z5	DESCRIPTION
SSP1	1750	500	1000		250		250 Z1 500 Z2 5 × (50 Z4/20" rest) 500 Z2 250 Z1
SSP2	2100	750	1000		350		250 Z1 500 Z2 7 × (50 Z4/20" rest) 500 Z2 500 Z1
SSP3	2500	1000	1000		500		500 Z1 500 Z2 10 × (50 Z4/20" rest) 500 Z2 500 Z1
SSP4	3100	1000	1500		600		500 Z1 500 Z2 12 × (50 Z4/20" rest) 1000 Z2 500 Z1
SSP5	1500	500	500		500		250 Z1 500 Z2 10 × (50 Z4/20" rest) 250 Z1
SSP6	1750	500	500		750		250 Z1 500 Z2 15 × (50 Z4/20" rest) 250 Z1
SSP7	1200	500	200		500		250 Z1 200 Z2 10 × (50 Z4/20" rest) 250 Z1

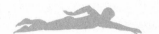

Time Trial and Taper Swims

Swim Time Trial and Swim Taper

Swim Time Trial (STT) and Swim Taper (STa)

The Swim Time Trial workout is built into many of our 80/20 triathlon training plans to provide an opportunity to reestablish zones and keep them current as your fitness increases through the training process. Feel free to use it for the same purpose outside the context of our readymade plans as an alternative to repeating the critical velocity test periodically.

The STa is designed for use within the prerace taper period, when the training workload is reduced to remove fatigue before competition and just enough hard work is included in the week to stay sharp.

STT and STa

CODE	DISTANCE	Z1	Z2	Z3	Z4	Z5	DESCRIPTION
STT1	1850	1250		600			250 Z1 400 Z3/120" rest 200 Z3/120" rest 1000 Z1
STT2	1000	400		600			200 Z1 400 Z3/120" rest 200 Z3/120" rest 200 Z1
STa1	1000	800		200			400 Z1 4 × (50 Z4/30" rest) 400 Z1

APPENDIX B:
80/20 CYCLING WORKOUTS

As noted in Chapter 8, the aggregate count of high intensity presented in the cycling and running workouts includes any recovery intervals of 3 minutes or less. For example, a segment of 3 × (5 min Z3/3 min Z1) would equal 24, not 15, minutes of Zone 3.

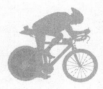

Low-Intensity Cycling Workouts

Cycling Recovery, Cycling Foundation, and Cycling Aerobic Intervals

Cycling Recovery (CRe)

Used sparingly in our 80/20 triathlon training plans, Cycling Recovery rides allow you to maintain fitness while regenerating for the next intense or long workout with a steady, gentle Zone 1 effort. Be wary of performing this workout in the context of a group ride, as it can be difficult to stay at the required intensity.

CRe

CODE	DURATION	Z1	Z2	Z3	Z4	Z5	DESCRIPTION
CRe1	20	20					20 min Z1
CRe2	25	25					25 min Z1
CRe3	30	30					30 min Z1
CRe4	35	35					35 min Z1
CRe5	40	40					40 min Z1
CRe6	45	45					45 min Z1
CRe7	50	50					50 min Z1
CRe8	55	55					55 min Z1
CRe9	60	60					60 min Z1
CRe10	75	75					75 min Z1
CRe11	90	90					90 min Z1
CRe12	105	105					105 min Z1
CRe13	120	120					120 min Z1
CRe14	150	150					150 min Z1

Cycling Foundation (CF)

Discipline and humility are demanded by the Cycling Foundation ride. One of the most frequently employed cycling workouts in all of our 80/20 triathlon training plans, it requires consistently correct execution if you are to succeed in maintaining the optimal 80/20 intensity balance. When done with fresh legs, there may be a strong temptation to drift above Zone 2. If you're competitive, swallow your pride and post these slow workouts on Strava anyway, saving your showoff efforts for the "20" of your 80/20 plan. Maintaining a high cadence (90 rpm or greater) will assist you in this objective.

CF

CODE	DURATION	Z1	Z2	Z3	Z4	Z5	DESCRIPTION
CF1	20	5	15				5 min in Z1 15 min Z2
CF2	25	10	15				5 min in Z1 15 min Z2 5 min Z1
CF3	30	10	20				5 min in Z1 20 min Z2 5 min Z1
CF4	35	10	25				5 min in Z1 25 min Z2 5 min Z1
CF5	40	10	30				5 min in Z1 30 min Z2 5 min Z1
CF6	45	10	35				5 min in Z1 35 min Z2 5 min Z1
CF7	50	10	40				5 min in Z1 40 min Z2 5 min Z1
CF8	55	10	45				5 min in Z1 45 min Z2 5 min Z1

(continues)

(Cycling Foundation continued)

CF

CODE	DURATION	Z1	Z2	Z3	Z4	Z5	DESCRIPTION
CF9	60	10	50				5 min in Z1 50 min Z2 5 min Z1
CF10	60	25	35				15 min in Z1 35 min Z2 10 min Z1
CF11	90	40	50				30 min in Z1 50 min Z2 10 min Z1
CF12	105	50	55				40 min in Z1 55 min Z2 10 min Z1
CF13	120	60	60				50 min in Z1 60 min Z2 10 min Z1
CF14	135	70	65				60 min in Z1 65 min Z2 10 min Z1
CF15	150	80	70				70 min in Z1 70 min Z2 10 min Z1
CF16	165	90	75				80 min in Z1 75 min Z2 10 min Z1
CF17	180	100	80				90 min in Z1 80 min Z2 10 min Z1
CF18	195	110	85				100 min in Z1 85 min Z2 10 min Z1
CF19	210	120	90				110 min in Z1 90 min Z2 10 min Z1

CF

CODE	DURATION	Z1	Z2	Z3	Z4	Z5	DESCRIPTION
CF20	225	130	95				120 min in Z1 95 min Z2 10 min Z1
CF21	240	140	100				130 min in Z1 100 min Z2 10 min Z1
CF22	270	150	120				140 min in Z1 120 min Z2 10 min Z1
CF23	300	160	140				150 min in Z1 140 min Z2 10 min Z1
CF24	330	170	160				160 min in Z1 160 min Z2 10 min Z1
CF25	360	180	180				170 min in Z1 180 min Z2 10 min Z1
CF26	75	10	65				5 min in Z1 65 min Z2 5 min Z1

Cycling Aerobic Intervals (CAe)

The Cycling Aerobic Interval ride serves primarily to prepare athletes for the specific intensity and stress of half and full Ironman racing. The Zone 2 intervals should be done at the expected intensity of your next long-distance race. For newer athletes, this will be toward the low end of Zone 2. More experienced triathlon cyclists will want to stay in the upper part of Zone 2, whereas highly advanced athletes may do these intervals in Zone X, which is technically moderate intensity, not low. In general, Sprint and Olympic athletes won't benefit from CAe workouts, though beginner triathletes sometimes benefit from limited use of CAe as preparation for more intense race-specific Zone 3 intervals.

CAe

CODE	DURATION	Z1	Z2	Z3	Z4	Z5	DESCRIPTION
CAe1	70	30	40				10 min Z1 2 × (20 min Z2/5 min Z1) 10 min Z1
CAe2	90	45	45				15 min Z1 3 × (15 min Z2/5 min Z1) 15 min Z1
CAe3	110	50	60				15 min Z1 4 × (15 min Z2/5 min Z1) 15 min Z1
CAe4	121	61	60				20 min Z1 3 × (20 min Z2/7 min Z1) 20 min Z1
CAe5	120	45	75				10 min Z1 5 × (15 min Z2/5 min Z1) 10 min Z1
CAe6	128	48	80				10 min Z1 4 × (20 min Z2/7 min Z1) 10 min Z1
CAe7	150	50	100				12 min Z1 4 × (25 min Z2/7 min Z1) 10 min Z1

CAe

CODE	DURATION	Z1	Z2	Z3	Z4	Z5	DESCRIPTION
CAe8	180	60	120				10 min Z1 4 × (30 min Z2/10 min Z1) 10 min Z1
CAe9	180	55	125				10 min Z1 5 × (25 min Z2/7 min Z1) 10 min Z1
CAe10	210	60	150				5 min Z1 5 × (30 min Z2/10 min Z1) 5 min Z1
CAe11	250	70	180				5 min Z1 6 × (30 min Z2/10 min Z1) 5 min Z1
CAe12	270	90	180				10 min Z1 6 × (30 min Z2/10 min Z1) 20 min Z1
CAe13	285	105	180				10 min Z1 6 × (30 min Z2/10 min Z1) 35 min Z1
CAe14	300	120	180				10 min Z1 6 × (30 min Z2/10 min Z1) 50 min Z1
CAe15	315	135	180				10 min Z1 6 × (30 min Z2/10 min Z1) 65 min Z1
CAe16	330	150	180				10 min Z1 6 × (30 min Z2/10 min Z1) 80 min Z1
CAe17	345	165	180				10 min Z1 6 × (30 min Z2/10 min Z1) 95 min Z1
CAe18	360	180	180				10 min Z1 6 × (30 min Z2/10 min Z1) 110 min Z1

(continues)

(Cycling Aerobic Intervals continued)

CAe

CODE	DURATION	Z1	Z2	Z3	Z4	Z5	DESCRIPTION
CAe19	210	90	120				10 min Z1 4 × (30 min Z2/10 min Z1) 40 min Z1
CAe20	240	120	120				10 min Z1 4 × (30 min Z2/10 min Z1) 70 min Z1
CAe21	270	150	120				10 min Z1 4 × (30 min Z2/10 min Z1) 100 min Z1
CAe22	300	180	120				10 min Z1 4 × (30 min Z2/10 min Z1) 130 min Z1
CAe23	330	210	120				10 min Z1 4 × (30 min Z2/10 min Z1) 160 min Z1
CAe24	360	240	120				10 min Z1 4 × (30 min Z2/10 min Z1) 190 min Z1
CAe25	390	270	120				10 min Z1 4 × (30 min Z2/10 min Z1) 220 min Z1
CAe26	420	300	120				10 min Z1 4 × (30 min Z2/10 min Z1) 250 min Z1
CAe27	240	13	227				10 min Z1 10 min Z2 3 × (4 min Z2/1 min Z1) 205 min Z2
CAe28	260	13	247				10 min Z1 10 min Z2 3 × (5 min Z2/1 min Z1) 222 min Z2

CAe

CODE	DURATION	Z1	Z2	Z3	Z4	Z5	DESCRIPTION
CAe29	280	13	267				10 min Z1 10 min Z2 3 × (6 min Z2/1 min Z1) 239 min Z2
CAe30	300	13	287				10 min Z1 10 min Z2 3 × (7 min Z2/1 min Z1) 256 min Z2
CAe31	320	13	307				10 min Z1 10 min Z2 3 × (8 min Z2/1 min Z1) 273 min Z2
CAe32	340	13	327				10 min Z1 10 min Z2 3 × (9 min Z2/1 min Z1) 290 min Z2
CAe33	360	13	347				10 min Z1 10 min Z2 3 × (10 min Z2/1 min Z1) 307 min Z2
CAe34	330	180	150				10 min Z1 5 × (30 min Z2/10 min Z1) 120 min Z1
CAe35	210	90	120				10 min Z1 4 × (30 min Z2/10 min Z1) 40 min Z1
CAe36	150	70	80				30 min Z1 4 × (20 min Z2/10 min Z1)
CAe37	165	85	80				30 min Z1 4 × (20 min Z2/10 min Z1) 15 min Z1

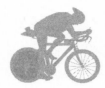

Moderate and High-Intensity Cycling

**Cycling Cruise Intervals, Cycling Tempo,
Cycling Fast Finish, Cycling Force, Cycling Mixed Intervals,
Cycling Anaerobic Intervals, Cycling Speed Play, and Bricks**

Cycling Cruise Intervals (CCI)

Muscular endurance is the ability to apply force over an extended period of time, and it is arguably the most important ability you can develop as a triathlete. No workout improves muscular endurance better than the Cruise Interval, which is the only interval workout type that is appropriate from the beginning to the end of a training cycle for all triathlon distances. Performed in Zone 3, Cruise Intervals should be executed at a very steady output from start to finish, regardless of their number or duration. Consider reducing the rest time from 3 minutes to 2 minutes and then from 2 minutes to 1 minute if you've mastered previous Cruise Interval rides to the point where you're tempted to stray above Zone 3.

CCI

CODE	DURATION	Z1	Z2	Z3	Z4	Z5	DESCRIPTION
CCI1	60	20	25	15			5 min Z1 20 min Z2 3 × (5 min Z3/3 min Z1) 5 min Z2 6 min Z1
CCI2	60	10	18	32			5 min Z1 5 min Z2 4 × (5 min Z3/3 min Z1) 13 min Z2 5 min Z1

CCI

CODE	DURATION	Z1	Z2	Z3	Z4	Z5	DESCRIPTION
CCI3	61	15	10	36			5 min Z1 10 min Z2 4 × (6 min Z3/3 min Z1) 5 min Z2 5 min Z1
CCI4	65	10	15	40			5 min Z1 10 min Z2 4 × (7 min Z3/3 min Z1) 5 min Z2 5 min Z1
CCI5	64	10	10	44			5 min Z1 5 min Z2 4 × (8 min Z3/3 min Z1) 5 min Z2 5 min Z1
CCI6	72	10	10	52			5 min Z1 5 min Z2 4 × (10 min Z3/3 min Z1) 5 min Z2 5 min Z1
CCI7	80	10	10	60			5 min Z1 5 min Z2 4 × (12 min Z3/3 min Z1) 5 min Z2 5 min Z1
CCI8	92	10	10	72			5 min Z1 5 min Z2 4 × (15 min Z3/3 min Z1) 5 min Z2 5 min Z1
CCI9	95	10	10	75			5 min Z1 5 min Z2 5 × (12 min Z3/3 min Z1) 5 min Z2 5 min Z1

(continues)

(Cycling Cruise Intervals continued)

CCI

CODE	DURATION	Z1	Z2	Z3	Z4	Z5	DESCRIPTION
CCI10	120	20	56	44			10 min Z1 15 min Z2 4 × (8 min Z3/3 min Z1) 40 min Z2 10 min Z1
CCI11	150	20	86	44			10 min Z1 15 min Z2 4 × (8 min Z3/3 min Z1) 71 min Z2 10 min Z1
CCI12	60	30	10	20			10 min Z1 10 min Z2 2 × (10 min Z3/4 min Z1) 12 min Z1
CCI13	90	15	39	36			10 min Z1 10 min Z2 4 × (6 min Z3/3 min Z1) 29 min Z2 5 min Z1
CCI14	90	15	35	40			10 min Z1 10 min Z2 4 × (7 min Z3/3 min Z1) 25 min Z2 5 min Z1
CCI15	90	15	31	44			10 min Z1 10 min Z2 4 × (8 min Z3/3 min Z1) 21 min Z2 5 min Z1
CCI16	90	15	27	48			10 min Z1 10 min Z2 4 × (9 min Z3/3 min Z1) 17 min Z2 5 min Z1
CCI17	30	15		15			10 min Z1 3 × (3 min Z3/2 min Z1) 5 min Z1

CCI

CODE	DURATION	Z1	Z2	Z3	Z4	Z5	DESCRIPTION
CCI18	105	15	54	36			10 min Z1 10 min Z2 4 × (6 min Z3/3 min Z1) 44 min Z2 5 min Z1
CCI19	120	25	59	36			20 min Z1 10 min Z2 4 × (6 min Z3/3 min Z1) 49 min Z2 5 min Z1
CCI20	90	10	48	32			5 min Z1 5 min Z2 4 × (5 min Z3/3 min Z1) 43 min Z2 5 min Z1
CCI21	90	50	20	20			10 min Z1 10 min Z2 2 × (10 min Z3/4 min Z1) 10 min Z2 32 min Z1
CCI22	90	25	50	15			10 min Z1 20 min Z2 3 × (3 min Z3/2 min Z1) 30 min Z2 15 min Z1
CCI23	91	20	50	21			10 min Z1 20 min Z2 3 × (5 min Z3/2 min Z1) 30 min Z2 10 min Z1
CCI24	121	20	80	21			10 min Z1 20 min Z2 3 × (5 min Z3/2 min Z1) 60 min Z2 10 min Z1

Cycling Tempo (CT)

The Cycling Tempo workout does an excellent job of developing muscular endurance and simulating Sprint and Olympic racing. The long duration of the Zone 3 segment makes the workout challenging and sensible pacing paramount. Start at the low end of Zone 3 and finish strong. A brief foray into Zone 4 at the end of the segment is acceptable. You may also use the CT to confirm or revise your 80/20 Zones for cycling by noting the point at which your heart rate plateaus during an extended period in upper Zone 3. (Recall the alternative LTHR test from page 63.)

CT

CODE	DURATION	Z1	Z2	Z3	Z4	Z5	DESCRIPTION
CT1	60	15	40	5			15 min Z1 5 min Z3 40 min Z2
CT2	35	10	10	15			5 min Z1 5 min Z2 15 min Z3 5 min Z2 5 min Z1
CT3	38	10	10	18			5 min Z1 5 min Z2 18 min Z3 5 min Z2 5 min Z1
CT4	40	10	10	20			5 min Z1 5 min Z2 20 min Z3 5 min Z2 5 min Z1
CT5	44	10	10	24			5 min Z1 5 min Z2 24 min Z3 5 min Z2 5 min Z1

CT

CODE	DURATION	Z1	Z2	Z3	Z4	Z5	DESCRIPTION
CT6	48	10	10	28			5 min Z1 5 min Z2 28 min Z3 5 min Z2 5 min Z1
CT7	50	10	10	30			5 min Z1 5 min Z2 30 min Z3 5 min Z2 5 min Z1
CT8	60	10	20	30			5 min Z1 10 min Z2 30 min Z3 10 min Z2 5 min Z1
CT9	75	10	45	20			5 min Z1 10 min Z2 20 min Z3 35 min Z2 5 min Z1
CT10	90	10	50	30			5 min Z1 10 min Z2 30 min Z3 40 min Z2 5 min Z1
CT11	105	10	75	20			5 min Z1 10 min Z2 20 min Z3 65 min Z2 5 min Z1
CT12	120	10	80	30			5 min Z1 10 min Z2 30 min Z3 70 min Z2 5 min Z1

(continues)

(Cycling Tempo continued)

CT

CODE	DURATION	Z1	Z2	Z3	Z4	Z5	DESCRIPTION
CT13	135	10	105	20			5 min Z1 10 min Z2 20 min Z3 95 min Z2 5 min Z1
CT14	150	10	110	30			5 min Z1 10 min Z2 30 min Z3 100 min Z2 5 min Z1
CT15	165	10	135	20			5 min Z1 10 min Z2 20 min Z3 125 min Z2 5 min Z1
CT16	180	10	140	30			5 min Z1 10 min Z2 30 min Z3 130 min Z2 5 min Z1
CT17	195	10	165	20			5 min Z1 10 min Z2 20 min Z3 155 min Z2 5 min Z1
CT18	210	10	170	30			5 min Z1 10 min Z2 30 min Z3 160 min Z2 5 min Z1
CT19	225	10	195	20			5 min Z1 10 min Z2 20 min Z3 185 min Z2 5 min Z1

CT

CODE	DURATION	Z1	Z2	Z3	Z4	Z5	DESCRIPTION
CT20	240	10	200	30			5 min Z1 10 min Z2 30 min Z3 190 min Z2 5 min Z1
CT21	255	10	225	20			5 min Z1 10 min Z2 20 min Z3 215 min Z2 5 min Z1
CT22	270	10	230	30			5 min Z1 10 min Z2 30 min Z3 220 min Z2 5 min Z1
CT23	285	10	255	20			5 min Z1 10 min Z2 20 min Z3 245 min Z2 5 min Z1
CT24	300	10	260	30			5 min Z1 10 min Z2 30 min Z3 250 min Z2 5 min Z1
CT25	52	10	10	32			5 min Z1 5 min Z2 32 min Z3 5 min Z2 5 min Z1
CT26	56	10	10	36			5 min Z1 5 min Z2 36 min Z3 5 min Z2 5 min Z1

(continues)

(Cycling Tempo continued)

CT

CODE	DURATION	Z1	Z2	Z3	Z4	Z5	DESCRIPTION
CT27	60	10	10	40			5 min Z1 5 min Z2 40 min Z3 5 min Z2 5 min Z1
CT28	65	10	10	45			5 min Z1 5 min Z2 45 min Z3 5 min Z2 5 min Z1
CT29	55	10	30	15			5 min Z1 15 min Z2 15 min Z3 15 min Z2 5 min Z1
CT30	60	10	30	20			5 min Z1 15 min Z2 20 min Z3 15 min Z2 5 min Z1
CT31	60	10	26	24			5 min Z1 15 min Z2 24 min Z3 11 min Z2 5 min Z1

Cycling Fast Finish (CFF)

One of the few workouts that positions the highest-intensity work at the end of the session with no subsequent cooldown, the Cycling Fast Finish ride cultivates the ability to ride hard on somewhat tired legs. Athletes tend to enjoy the CFF, reporting that the concluding Zone 3 surge feels like a reward for holding back to Zone 2 during the bulk of the ride.

CFF

CODE	DURATION	Z1	Z2	Z3	Z4	Z5	DESCRIPTION
CFF1	25	5	15	5			5 min Z1 15 min Z2 5 min Z3
CFF2	30	5	20	5			5 min Z1 20 min Z2 5 min Z3
CFF3	30	5	15	10			5 min Z1 15 min Z2 10 min Z3
CFF4	40	5	25	10			5 min Z1 25 min Z2 10 min Z3
CFF5	42	5	25	12			5 min Z1 25 min Z2 12 min Z3
CFF6	47	5	30	12			5 min Z1 30 min Z2 12 min Z3
CFF7	52	5	35	12			5 min Z1 35 min Z2 12 min Z3
CFF8	55	5	35	15			5 min Z1 35 min Z2 15 min Z3

(continues)

(Cycling Fast Finish continued)

CFF

CODE	DURATION	Z1	Z2	Z3	Z4	Z5	DESCRIPTION
CFF9	60	5	40	15			5 min Z1 40 min Z2 15 min Z3
CFF10	65	5	45	15			5 min Z1 45 min Z2 15 min Z3
CFF11	75	5	55	15			5 min Z1 55 min Z2 15 min Z3
CFF12	90	5	70	15			5 min Z1 70 min Z2 15 min Z3
CFF13	105	5	85	15			5 min Z1 85 min Z2 15 min Z3
CFF14	120	5	100	15			5 min Z1 100 min Z2 15 min Z3
CFF15	135	5	115	15			5 min Z1 115 min Z2 15 min Z3
CFF16	150	5	130	15			5 min Z1 130 min Z2 15 min Z3
CFF17	165	5	145	15			5 min Z1 145 min Z2 15 min Z3
CFF18	180	5	160	15			5 min Z1 160 min Z2 15 min Z3
CFF19	195	5	175	15			5 min Z1 175 min Z2 15 min Z3

CFF

CODE	DURATION	Z1	Z2	Z3	Z4	Z5	DESCRIPTION
CFF20	210	5	190	15			5 min Z1 190 min Z2 15 min Z3
CFF21	225	5	205	15			5 min Z1 205 min Z2 15 min Z3
CFF22	240	5	220	15			5 min Z1 220 min Z2 15 min Z3
CFF23	270	5	250	15			5 min Z1 250 min Z2 15 min Z3
CFF24	300	5	280	15			5 min Z1 280 min Z2 15 min Z3
CFF25	330	5	310	15			5 min Z1 310 min Z2 15 min Z3
CFF26	360	5	340	15			5 min Z1 340 min Z2 15 min Z3
CFF27	60	5	45	10			5 min Z1 45 min Z2 10 min Z3

Cycling Force (CFo)

A terrific builder of pedaling efficiency and power, the Cycling Force ride offers an excellent opportunity to go very hard, but be sure to complete each uphill interval with a similar output and avoid fading near the end. Because the intervals are so short, it is necessary to use power or perceived effort to gauge intensity in this session, as heart rate is unlikely to reach Zone 5 prior to the end of each interval. No hills? No problem; you can simulate them by riding in a high gear, reducing your cadence to 65–75 rpm, and pedaling occasionally from a standing position.

CFo

CODE	DURATION	Z1	Z2	Z3	Z4	Z5	DESCRIPTION
CFo1	27	10	5			12	5 min Z1 5 min Z2 6 × (30" Z5/90" Z1) 5 min Z1
CFo2	31	10	5			16	5 min Z1 5 min Z2 8 × (30" Z5/90" Z1) 5 min Z1
CFo3	33	10	5			18	5 min Z1 5 min Z2 6 × (1 min Z5/2 min Z1) 5 min Z1
CFo4	35	10	5			20	5 min Z1 5 min Z2 10 × (30" Z5/90" Z1) 5 min Z1
CFo5	39	10	5			24	5 min Z1 5 min Z2 12 × (30" Z5/90" Z1) 5 min Z1
CFo6	39	10	5			24	5 min Z1 5 min Z2 8 × (1 min Z5/2 min Z1) 5 min Z1

CFo

CODE	DURATION	Z1	Z2	Z3	Z4	Z5	DESCRIPTION
CFo7	39	10	5			24	5 min Z1 5 min Z2 6 × (1.5 min Z5/2.5 min Z1) 5 min Z1
CFo8	45	10	5			30	5 min Z1 5 min Z2 10 × (1 min Z5/2 min Z1) 5 min Z1
CFo9	47	10	5			32	5 min Z1 5 min Z2 8 × (1.5 min Z5/2.5 min Z1) 5 min Z1
CFo10	51	10	5			36	5 min Z1 5 min Z2 12 × (1 min Z5/2 min Z1) 5 min Z1
CFo11	55	10	5			40	5 min Z1 5 min Z2 10 × (1.5 min Z5/2.5 min Z1) 5 min Z1
CFo12	63	10	5			48	5 min Z1 5 min Z2 12 × (1.5 min Z5/2.5 min Z1) 5 min Z1
CFo13	70	10	20			40	5 min Z1 10 min Z2 10 × (1.5 min Z5/2.5 min Z1) 10 min Z2 5 min Z1
CFo14	135	20	85			30	15 min Z1 15 min Z2 10 × (1 min Z5/2 min Z1) 70 min Z2 5 min Z1

(continues)

(Cycling Force continued)

CFo

CODE	DURATION	Z1	Z2	Z3	Z4	Z5	DESCRIPTION
CFo15	150	20	100			30	15 min Z1 15 min Z2 10 × (1 min Z5/2 min Z1) 85 min Z2 5 min Z1
CFo16	180	20	130			30	15 min Z1 15 min Z2 10 × (1 min Z5/2 min Z1) 115 min Z2 5 min Z1
CFo17	74	10	40			24	5 min Z1 5 min Z2 12 × (30" Z5/90" Z1) 35 min Z2 5 min Z1
CFo18	78	50	10			18	5 min Z1 10 min Z2 6 × (1 min Z5/2 min Z1) 40 min Z2 5 min Z1
CFo19	90	61	5			24	5 min Z1 15 min Z2 8 × (1 min Z5/2 min Z1) 46 min Z2
CFo20	165	15	120			30	10 min Z1 15 min Z2 10 × (1 min Z5/2 min Z1) 105 min Z2 5 min Z1
CFo21	120	20	70			30	15 min Z1 15 min Z2 10 × (1 min Z5/2 min Z1) 55 min Z2 5 min Z1

CFo

CODE	DURATION	Z1	Z2	Z3	Z4	Z5	DESCRIPTION
CFo22	60	38	10			12	10 min Z1 10 min Z2 8 × (30" Z5/60" Z1) 28 min Z1
CFo23	105	20	55			30	15 min Z1 15 min Z2 10 × (1 min Z5/2 min Z1) 40 min Z2 5 min Z1
CFo24	90	35	40			15	15 min Z1 15 min Z2 5 × (1 min Z5/2 min Z1) 25 min Z2 20 min Z1

Cycling Mixed Intervals (CMI)

The Cycling Mixed Intervals ride is an exceptionally challenging workout designed to increase lactate threshold and aerobic capacity. Half and full Ironman athletes may question the necessity of the suffering caused by this session, but the raw increase in sustainable output that results from it will pay off in subsequent workouts and on race day. Whereas athletes training for longer triathlons need not incorporate CMIs into their training beyond the midpoint of a training cycle, sprint and Olympic-distance racers should sprinkle them throughout it. Pacing is critical in the first Zone 3 interval; start at the low end of the zone and work your way up.

CMI

CODE	DURATION	Z1	Z2	Z3	Z4	Z5	DESCRIPTION
CMI1	120	50		40	30		20 min Z1 2 × (20 min Z3/15 min Z1) 10 × (1 min Z4/2 min Z1)
CMI2	150	80		40	30		20 min Z1 2 × (20 min Z3/15 min Z1) 10 × (1 min Z4/2 min Z1) 30 min Z1
CMI3	165	95		40	30		20 min Z1 2 × (20 min Z3/15 min Z1) 10 × (1 min Z4/2 min Z1) 45 min Z1
CMI4	180	110		40	30		20 min Z1 2 × (20 min Z3/15 min Z1) 10 × (1 min Z4/2 min Z1) 60 min Z1
CMI5	210	140		40	30		20 min Z1 2 × (20 min Z3/15 min Z1) 10 × (1 min Z4/2 min Z1) 90 min Z1
CMI6	120	65		40	15		20 min Z1 2 × (20 min Z3/15 min Z1) 5 × (1 min Z4/2 min Z1) 15 min Z1

Cycling Anaerobic Intervals (CAn)

When executed properly, the Cycling Anaerobic Interval ride is the most effective way to increase your aerobic capacity, or VO_2max. While VO_2max is widely overrated as the be-all and end-all of endurance fitness, an increase in aerobic capacity almost always translates to better race performance. Additionally, intervals performed at an intensity that elicits VO_2max (namely, Zone 4) are proven to be more effective at improving overall movement economy than either Zone 3 or Zone 5 intervals. Successful integration of these intervals into the early phase of training places you in an advantageous position leading up to your race. Make no mistake: CAn workouts are challenging. Take great care to do these intervals neither too slow nor too fast (in other words, stay away from Zone 3 or Zone 5 intensity). The comparatively long rest period between intervals reflects the difficulty of the Zone 4 work.

CAn

CODE	DURATION	Z1	Z2	Z3	Z4	Z5	DESCRIPTION
CAn1	60	50			10		15 min Z1 4 × (2.5 min Z4/5 min Z1) 15 min Z1
CAn2	62.5	50			12.5		15 min Z1 5 × (2.5 min Z4/5 min Z1) 10 min Z1
CAn3	60	45			15		10 min Z1 6 × (2.5 min Z4/5 min Z1) 5 min Z1
CAn4	90	45	30		15		10 min Z1 6 × (2.5 min Z4/5 min Z1) 30 min Z2 5 min Z1
CAn5	120	45	60		15		10 min Z1 6 × (2.5 min Z4/5 min Z1) 60 min Z2 5 min Z1

(continues)

(Cycling Anaerobic Intervals continued)

CAn

CODE	DURATION	Z1	Z2	Z3	Z4	Z5	DESCRIPTION
CAn6	150	45	90		15		10 min Z1 10 min Z2 6 × (2.5 min Z4/5 min Z1) 80 min Z2 5 min Z1
CAn7	92.5	20	65		7.5		10 min Z1 10 min Z2 3 × (2.5 min Z4/5 min Z1) 45 min Z2 5 min Z1
CAn8	150	35	105		10		10 min Z1 10 min Z2 4 × (2.5 min Z4/5 min Z1) 95 min Z2 5 min Z1
CAn9	60	40	12		8		10 min Z1 10 min Z2 3 × (2.5 min Z4/5 min Z1) 17 min Z1

Cycling Speed Play (CSP)

Similar in format to the Zone 5 Cycling Force ride, the Cycling Speed Play ride features longer Zone 4 intervals with shorter recoveries. The big mistake to avoid when executing this workout is pushing too hard (Zone 5), which will cause you to fade and fail to complete the interval at the appropriate intensity. Be sure also to perform the CSP in a seated position.

CSP

CODE	DURATION	Z1	Z2	Z3	Z4	Z5	DESCRIPTION
CSP1	27	10	5		12		5 min Z1 5 min Z2 3 × (2 min Z4/2 min Z1) 5 min Z1
CSP2	60	10	35		15		5 min Z1 5 min Z2 5 × (1 min Z4/2 min Z1) 30 min Z2 5 min Z1
CSP3	31	10	5		16		5 min Z1 5 min Z2 4 × (2 min Z4/2 min Z1) 5 min Z1
CSP4	60	10	32		18		5 min Z1 5 min Z2 6 × (1 min Z4/2 min Z1) 27 min Z2 5 min Z1
CSP5	35	10	5		20		5 min Z1 5 min Z2 5 × (2 min Z4/2 min Z1) 5 min Z1
CSP6	60	10	29		21		5 min Z1 5 min Z2 7 × (1 min Z4/2 min Z1) 30 min Z2 5 min Z1

(continues)

(Cycling Speed Play continued)

CSP

CODE	DURATION	Z1	Z2	Z3	Z4	Z5	DESCRIPTION
CSP7	39	10	5		24		5 min Z1 5 min Z2 6 × (2 min Z4/2 min Z1) 5 min Z1
CSP8	60	10	26		24		5 min Z1 5 min Z2 8 × (1 min Z4/2 min Z1) 26 min Z2
CSP9	42	10	5		27		5 min Z1 5 min Z2 9 × (1 min Z4/2 min Z1) 5 min Z1
CSP10	60	10	22		28		5 min Z1 5 min Z2 7 × (2 min Z4/2 min Z1) 17 min Z2 5 min Z1
CSP11	45	10	5		30		5 min Z1 5 min Z2 10 × (1 min Z4/2 min Z1) 5 min Z1
CSP12	60	10	18		32		5 min Z1 5 min Z2 8 × (2 min Z4/2 min Z1) 13 min Z2 5 min Z1
CSP13	51	10	5		36		5 min Z1 5 min Z2 9 × (2 min Z4/2 min Z1) 5 min Z1

CSP

CODE	DURATION	Z1	Z2	Z3	Z4	Z5	DESCRIPTION
CSP14	61	10	15		36		5 min Z1 5 min Z2 12 × (1 min Z4/2 min Z1) 10 min Z2 5 min Z1
CSP15	79	25	30		24		10 min Z1 15 min Z2 6 × (2 min Z4/2 min Z1) 15 min Z2 15 min Z1
CSP16	87	25	30		32		10 min Z1 15 min Z2 8 × (2 min Z4/2 min Z1) 15 min Z2 15 min Z1
CSP17	79	25	30		24		10 min Z1 15 min Z2 8 × (1 min Z4/2 min Z1) 15 min Z2 15 min Z1
CSP18	90	36	30		24		21 min Z1 15 min Z2 8 × (1 min Z4/2 min Z1) 15 min Z2 15 min Z1

Brick (BR)

Reserved for the final weeks before a Sprint or Olympic race, the Brick workout is pure race simulation. Long, intense Zone 3 intervals are the best dress rehearsal for race day. Whereas in a traditional brick workout the bike and run segments are completed separately (with the run typically taking place after the bike ride), our 80/20 brick intervals oscillate from bike to run and back again two or more times. This structure avoids a common situation where the run portion of the brick is performed exclusively on fatigued legs, limiting the running fitness that can be gained from the workout. The frequent switches from one discipline to the other will also help you master the transition between cycling and running, an overlooked part of triathlon racing where precious seconds can be gained or lost.

Sprint athletes should perform the intervals at the upper end of Zone 3, Olympic racers at the lower end of Zone 3, and the beginner BR1 and BR2 intervals at the upper end of Zone 2 for all distances. If you are an orthodox triathlete who can't fathom cycling after running, you can disregard the oscillating nature of this version of the brick and perform all the bike intervals before the run intervals. Half and full Ironman athletes will use the weekend CAe workouts for their bricks as discussed in Chapters 11 and 12.

The Brick workout descriptions are complicated enough to merit a closer inspection. Let's look at the BR3 as an example:

Bike 15 min Z1, 2 × (Run 7 min Z3/3 min Z1 → Bike 10 min Z3/3 min Z1), 5 min Z1

The first phrase, "Bike 15 min Z1," is, as usual, your warm-up.

"2 × (Run 7 min Z3/3 min Z1 → Bike 10 min Z3/3 min Z1)" looks complicated, but it won't feel that way the first time you perform the workout. You'll start this segment by running for 7 minutes in Zone 3 and then for 3 minutes in Zone 1. These minutes can include your transition from run to bike gear, after which you will bike for 10 minutes in Zone 3, then spend 3 minutes recovering and transitioning back to the run. You'll repeat this sequence two times. Note that the → symbol represents the quick transition from running to cycling.

"5 min Z1" is your well-deserved cooldown.

BR

CODE	DURATION	Z1	Z2	Z3	Z4	Z5	DESCRIPTION
BR1	90	30	60				Bike 20 min Z1 2 × (Run 10 min Z2 → Bike 20 min Z2) 10 min Z1
BR2	120	30	90				Bike 20 min Z1 3 × (Run 10 min Z2 → Bike 20 min Z2) 10 min Z1
BR3	61	15		46			Bike 15 min Z1 2 × (Run 7 min Z3/3 min Z1 → Bike 10 min Z3/3 min Z1)
BR4	89	20		69			Bike 15 min Z1 3 × (Run 7 min Z3/3 min Z1 → Bike 10 min Z3/3 min Z1) 5 min Z1
BR5	112	20		92			Bike 15 min Z1 4 × (Run 7 min Z3/3 min Z1 → Bike 10 min Z3/3 min Z1) 5 min Z1
BR6	135	20		115			Bike 15 min Z1 5 × (Run 7 min Z3/3 min Z1 → Bike 10 min Z3/3 min Z1) 5 min Z1

APPENDIX C:
80/20 RUNNING WORKOUTS

Low-Intensity Runs

Running Recovery, Running Foundation, and Running Aerobic Intervals

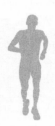

Running Recovery (RRe)

"Running Recovery" is a bit of a misnomer. Jogging in Zone 1 will not actually accelerate your recovery from a prior hard workout. It will, however, give you a gentle aerobic training stimulus without inhibiting recovery from a prior hard workout. Pay especially close attention to your intensity when doing this session, stay in Zone 1 no matter how slowly you have to go to do so, and save your energy for the more intense workout around the corner.

RRe

CODE	DURATION	Z1	Z2	Z3	Z4	Z5	DESCRIPTION
RRe1	20	20					20 min Z1
RRe2	25	25					25 min Z1
RRe3	30	30					30 min Z1
RRe4	35	35					35 min Z1
RRe5	40	40					40 min Z1
RRe6	45	45					45 min Z1
RRe7	50	50					50 min Z1
RRe8	55	55					55 min Z1
RRe9	60	60					60 min Z1

Running Foundation (RF)

The basic aerobic run, which we call Running Foundation, is the most commonly botched workout in the sport of triathlon. Meant to be done at least slightly below the ventilatory threshold, it is typically done above it. Counterintuitive though it may be, consistently holding yourself back in this critical bread-and-butter workout may do more to help you improve as a triathlete than any other change you make to your training. Consider Zone 2 the "vegetables" of your training diet. Whether you hate or love the intensity, a healthy dose nourishes long-term rewards.

RF

CODE	DURATION	Z1	Z2	Z3	Z4	Z5	DESCRIPTION
RF1	20	10	10				5 min in Z1 10 min Z2 5 min Z1
RF2	25	10	15				5 min in Z1 15 min Z2 5 min Z1
RF3	30	10	20				5 min in Z1 20 min Z2 5 min Z1
RF4	35	10	25				5 min in Z1 25 min Z2 5 min Z1
RF5	40	10	30				5 min in Z1 30 min Z2 5 min Z1
RF6	45	10	35				5 min in Z1 35 min Z2 5 min Z1
RF7	50	10	40				5 min in Z1 40 min Z2 5 min Z1

RF

CODE	DURATION	Z1	Z2	Z3	Z4	Z5	DESCRIPTION
RF8	55	10	45				5 min in Z1 45 min Z2 5 min Z1
RF9	60	10	50				5 min in Z1 50 min Z2 5 min Z1
RF10	70	10	60				5 min in Z1 60 min Z2 5 min Z1
RF11	80	10	70				5 min in Z1 70 min Z2 5 min Z1
RF12	90	10	80				5 min in Z1 80 min Z2 5 min Z1
RF13	70	10	60				5 min in Z1 60 min Z2 5 min Z1
RF14	100	10	90				5 min in Z1 90 min Z2 5 min Z1
RF15	110	10	100				5 min in Z1 100 min Z2 5 min Z1
RF16	105	10	95				5 min in Z1 95 min Z2 5 min Z1
RF17	120	10	110				5 min in Z1 110 min Z2 5 min Z1

Running Aerobic Intervals (RAe)

With few exceptions, the Running Aerobic Intervals workout is reserved for half and full Ironman training. The Zone 2 intervals should be done at the expected intensity of your next half or full Ironman. If you're relatively new to the sport, aim for the lower end of Zone 2. More experienced athletes can settle into the upper end of Zone 2. The most advanced competitors may need to cross over into Zone X to reach race intensity. In general, sprint and Olympic athletes won't benefit from RAe workouts, although beginners may use RAe workouts as preparation for the more intense race-specific Zone 3 intervals.

RAe

CODE	DURATION	Z1	Z2	Z3	Z4	Z5	DESCRIPTION
RAe1	60	30	30				10 min Z1 3 × (10 min Z2/3 min Z1) 11 min Z1
RAe2	90	60	30				15 min Z1 3 × (10 min Z2/3 min Z1) 36 min Z1
RAe3	75	35	40				12 min Z1 4 × (10 min Z2/3 min Z1) 11 min Z1
RAe4	90	45	45				15 min Z1 3 × (15 min Z2/5 min Z1) 15 min Z1
RAe5	90	30	60				10 min Z1 4 × (15 min Z2/5 min Z1)
RAe6	105	45	60				10 min Z1 4 × (15 min Z2/5 min Z1) 15 min Z1
RAe7	120	60	60				10 min Z1 4 × (15 min Z2/5 min Z1) 30 min Z1

RAe

CODE	DURATION	Z1	Z2	Z3	Z4	Z5	DESCRIPTION
RAe8	135	75	60				10 min Z1 4 × (15 min Z2/5 min Z1) 45 min Z1
RAe9	150	90	60				10 min Z1 4 × (15 min Z2/5 min Z1) 60 min Z1
RAe10	105	60	45				10 min Z1 3 × (15 min Z2/5 min Z1) 35 min Z1
RAe11	120	75	45				10 min Z1 3 × (15 min Z2/5 min Z1) 50 min Z1
RAe12	135	90	45				10 min Z1 3 × (15 min Z2/5 min Z1) 65 min Z1
RAe13	150	105	45				10 min Z1 3 × (15 min Z2/5 min Z1) 80 min Z1
RAe14	120	13	107				10 min Z1 3 × (4 min Z2/1 min Z1) 95 min Z2
RAe15	130	13	117				10 min Z1 3 × (5 min Z2/1 min Z1) 102 min Z2
RAe16	140	13	127				10 min Z1 3 × (6 min Z2/1 min Z1) 109 min Z2
RAe17	150	13	137				10 min Z1 3 × (7 min Z2/1 min Z1) 116 min Z2
RAe18	160	13	147				10 min Z1 3 × (8 min Z2/1 min Z1) 123 min Z2

(continues)

(Running Aerobic Intervals continued)

RAe

CODE	DURATION	Z1	Z2	Z3	Z4	Z5	DESCRIPTION
RAe19	170	13	157				10 min Z1 3 × (9 min Z2/1 min Z1) 130 min Z2
RAe20	180	13	167				10 min Z1 3 × (10 min Z2/1 min Z1) 137 min Z2
RAe21	165	14	151				10 min Z1 4 × (15 min Z2/1 min Z1) 90 min Z2
RAe22	46	16	30				10 min Z1 3 × (10 min Z2/2 min Z1)

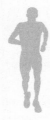

Moderate and High-Intensity Running

Running Cruise Intervals, Running Tempo, Running Fast Finish, Running Hill Repeats, Running Mixed Intervals, Running Anaerobic Intervals, Running Short Intervals, Running Speed Play, and Run Taper

Running Cruise Intervals (RCI)

The Running Cruise Interval workout is another bread-and-butter session that should have a place in your routine no matter which competitive distance you're preparing for or where you are in the training cycle. As a Zone 3 workout, it is done at or near your lactate threshold pace. Practicing this pace will enable you to maintain it longer and more efficiently and thereby achieve faster triathlon run splits. Consider reducing the rest time from 3 minutes to as little as 1 minute if previous Cruise Intervals sets have been successful.

RCI

CODE	DURATION	Z1	Z2	Z3	Z4	Z5	DESCRIPTION
RCI1	60	10	26	24			5 min Z1 21 min Z2 3 × (5 min Z3/3 min Z1) 5 min Z2 5 min Z1
RCI2	52	10	10	32			5 min Z1 5 min Z2 4 × (5 min Z3/3 min Z1) 5 min Z2 5 min Z1
RCI3	64	10	10	44			5 min Z1 5 min Z2 4 × (8 min Z3/3 min Z1) 5 min Z2 5 min Z1
RCI4	72	10	10	52			5 min Z1 5 min Z2 4 × (10 min Z3/3 min Z1) 5 min Z2 5 min Z1
RCI5	80	10	10	60			5 min Z1 5 min Z2 4 × (12 min Z3/3 min Z1) 5 min Z2 5 min Z1
RCI6	92	10	10	72			5 min Z1 5 min Z2 4 × (15 min Z3/3 min Z1) 5 min Z2 5 min Z1

(*continues*)

(Running Cruise Intervals continued)

RCI

CODE	DURATION	Z1	Z2	Z3	Z4	Z5	DESCRIPTION
RCI7	70	22	28	20			15 min Z1 11 min Z2 2 × (10 min Z3/4 min Z1) 11 min Z2 5 min Z1
RCI8	70	10	24	36			5 min Z1 10 min Z2 4 × (6 min Z3/3 min Z1) 14 min Z2 5 min Z1
RCI9	74	10	24	40			5 min Z1 10 min Z2 4 × (7 min Z3/3 min Z1) 14 min Z2 5 min Z1
RCI10	45	10	11	24			5 min Z1 6 min Z2 3 × (6 min Z3/2 min Z1) 5 min Z2 5 min Z1
RCI11	53	10	11	32			5 min Z1 6 min Z2 4 × (6 min Z3/2 min Z1) 5 min Z2 5 min Z1
RCI12	61	10	15	36			5 min Z1 10 min Z2 4 × (7 min Z3/2 min Z1) 5 min Z2 5 min Z1

RCI

CODE	DURATION	Z1	Z2	Z3	Z4	Z5	DESCRIPTION
RCI13	30	15		15			10 min Z1 3 × (3 min Z3/2 min Z1) 5 min Z1
RCI14	71	21	10	40			5 min Z1 10 min Z2 4 × (10 min Z3/4 min Z1)
RCI15	38	15	5	18			15 min Z1 3 × (4 min Z3/2 min Z1) 5 min Z2

Running Tempo (RT)

The Running Tempo workout serves two purposes. First, it simulates the intensity and duration of sprint and Olympic racing. Second, it affords an opportunity to verify lactate threshold using one of the alternative testing methods described in Chapter 6. For example, as the RT3 version of the workout prescribes 20 minutes in Zone 3, you could take your average pace performing that segment at upper Zone 3, and multiply it by 0.95 to get an estimate of your current threshold pace. Or, if you find the RT1 version on your schedule, you can watch your heart rate during the fifteen-minute Z3 effort, note when it levels off, and use this number as your LTHR going forward.

RT

CODE	DURATION	Z1	Z2	Z3	Z4	Z5	DESCRIPTION
RT1	35	10	10	15			5 min Z1 5 min Z2 15 min Z3 5 min Z2 5 min Z1
RT2	38	10	10	18			5 min Z1 5 min Z2 18 min Z3 5 min Z2 5 min Z1
RT3	40	10	10	20			5 min Z1 5 min Z2 20 min Z3 5 min Z2 5 min Z1
RT4	44	10	10	24			5 min Z1 5 min Z2 24 min Z3 5 min Z2 5 min Z1

RT

CODE	DURATION	Z1	Z2	Z3	Z4	Z5	DESCRIPTION
RT5	48	10	10	28			5 min Z1 5 min Z2 28 min Z3 5 min Z2 5 min Z1
RT6	50	10	10	30			5 min Z1 5 min Z2 30 min Z3 5 min Z2 5 min Z1
RT7	52	10	10	32			5 min Z1 5 min Z2 32 min Z3 5 min Z2 5 min Z1
RT8	56	10	10	36			5 min Z1 5 min Z2 36 min Z3 5 min Z2 5 min Z1
RT9	60	10	10	40			5 min Z1 5 min Z2 40 min Z3 5 min Z2 5 min Z1
RT10	65	10	10	45			5 min Z1 5 min Z2 45 min Z3 5 min Z2 5 min Z1

(*continues*)

(Running Tempo continued)

RT

CODE	DURATION	Z1	Z2	Z3	Z4	Z5	DESCRIPTION
RT11	50	10	30	10			5 min Z1 15 min Z2 10 min Z3 15 min Z2 5 min Z1
RT12	55	10	35	10			5 min Z1 15 min Z2 10 min Z3 20 min Z2 5 min Z1
RT13	50	10	20	20			5 min Z1 10 min Z2 20 min Z3 10 min Z2 5 min Z1
RT14	54	10	20	24			5 min Z1 10 min Z2 24 min Z3 10 min Z2 5 min Z1
RT15	62	10	20	32			5 min Z1 10 min Z2 32 min Z3 10 min Z2 5 min Z1
RT16	60	20	20	20			10 min Z1 10 min Z2 20 min Z3 10 min Z2 10 min Z1

RT

CODE	DURATION	Z1	Z2	Z3	Z4	Z5	DESCRIPTION
RT17	76	20	20	36			10 min Z1 10 min Z2 36 min Z3 10 min Z2 10 min Z1
RT18	70	10	20	40			5 min Z1 10 min Z2 40 min Z3 10 min Z2 5 min Z1
RT19	90	10	60	20			5 min Z1 10 min Z2 20 min Z3 50 min Z2 5 min Z1
RT20	90	55	10	25			5 min Z1 10 min Z2 25 min Z3 50 min Z1

Running Fast Finish (RFF)

Developing the ability to run fast when fatigued is a crucial part of triathlon run training. The Running Fast Finish workout does the job better than any other, with the possible exception of certain bike/run brick sessions.

RFF

CODE	DURATION	Z1	Z2	Z3	Z4	Z5	DESCRIPTION
RFF1	25	5	15	5			5 min Z1 15 min Z2 5 min Z3
RFF2	30	5	20	5			5 min Z1 20 min Z2 5 min Z3
RFF3	35	5	20	10			5 min Z1 20 min Z2 10 min Z3
RFF4	40	5	25	10			5 min Z1 25 min Z2 10 min Z3
RFF5	42	5	25	12			5 min Z1 25 min Z2 12 min Z3
RFF6	47	5	30	12			5 min Z1 30 min Z2 12 min Z3
RFF7	52	5	35	12			5 min Z1 35 min Z2 12 min Z3

RFF

CODE	DURATION	Z1	Z2	Z3	Z4	Z5	DESCRIPTION
RFF8	55	5	35	15			5 min Z1 35 min Z2 15 min Z3
RFF9	60	5	40	15			5 min Z1 40 min Z2 15 min Z3
RFF10	65	5	45	15			5 min Z1 45 min Z2 15 min Z3
RFF11	60	5	45	10			5 min Z1 45 min Z2 10 min Z3

Running Hill Repeats (RHR)

The Running Hill Repeats workout will add power and efficiency to your stride. Because the Zone 5 efforts at the core of the session are so short, you will have to use pace, power, or perceived effort to gauge intensity, as your heart rate may not reach Zone 5 before the end of each ascent. If you like to run hard, this workout is an excellent opportunity to do so, but avoid running so hard that you cannot complete all of the prescribed hill repeats at the same output. If hills are difficult or impossible to access in your area, do the RHR on a treadmill with the belt set at an incline of 6 to 8 percent. If you don't have access to a treadmill either, run your Zone 5 intervals on a flat surface. (See Running Short Intervals (RSI), which can be used in place of the RHR when no gradient can be found.)

RHR

CODE	DURATION	Z1	Z2	Z3	Z4	Z5	DESCRIPTION
RHR1	45	5	32			8	5 min Z1 32 min Z2 4 × (30" Z5 uphill/90" Z1)
RHR2	27	10	5			12	5 min Z1 5 min Z2 6 × (30" Z5 uphill/90" Z1) 5 min Z1
RHR3	31	10	5			16	5 min Z1 5 min Z2 8 × (30" Z5 uphill/90" Z1) 5 min Z1
RHR4	33	10	5			18	5 min Z1 5 min Z2 6 × (1 min Z5 uphill/2 min Z1) 5 min Z1
RHR5	35	10	5			20	5 min Z1 5 min Z2 10 × (30" Z5 uphill/90" Z1) 5 min Z1
RHR6	39	10	5			24	5 min Z1 5 min Z2 12 × (30" Z5 uphill/90" Z1) 5 min Z1

RHR

CODE	DURATION	Z1	Z2	Z3	Z4	Z5	DESCRIPTION
RHR7	39	10	5			24	5 min Z1 5 min Z2 8 × (1 min Z5 uphill/2 min Z1) 5 min Z1
RHR8	39	10	5			24	5 min Z1 5 min Z2 6 × (1.5 min Z5 uphill/2.5 min Z1) 5 min Z1
RHR9	45	10	5			30	5 min Z1 5 min Z2 10 × (1 min Z5 uphill/2 min Z1) 5 min Z1
RHR10	47	10	5			32	5 min Z1 5 min Z2 8 × (1.5 min Z5 uphill/2.5 min Z1) 5 min Z1
RHR11	51	10	5			36	5 min Z1 5 min Z2 12 × (1 min Z5 uphill/2 min Z1) 5 min Z1
RHR12	55	10	5			40	5 min Z1 5 min Z2 10 × (1.5 min Z5 uphill/2.5 min Z1) 5 min Z1
RHR13	63	10	5			48	5 min Z1 5 min Z2 12 × (1.5 min Z5 uphill/2.5 min Z1) 5 min Z1
RHR14	50	10	20			20	5 min Z1 20 min Z2 10 × (30" Z5 uphill/90" Z1) 5 min Z1

Running Mixed Intervals (RMI)

Complex in execution, the Running Mixed Intervals workout offers rewards to match. As the only workout to span the gamut from Zone 1 to 5, this session requires some study and planning prior to execution. You should feel a high level of discomfort during this workout, but if you reach the agony stage it is time to back off. Remember, pain is temporary, but your official run split on the Internet is forever!

RMI

CODE	DURATION	Z1	Z2	Z3	Z4	Z5	DESCRIPTION
RMI1	36	18	5	5	6	2	5 min Z1 5 min Z2 1 min Z5 2 min Z1 3 min Z4 2 min Z1 5 min Z3 2 min Z1 3 min Z4 2 min Z1 1 min Z5 5 min Z1
RMI2	46	18	5	10	10	3	5 min Z1 5 min Z2 1.5 min Z5 2 min Z1 5 min Z4 2 min Z1 10 min Z3 2 min Z1 5 min Z4 2 min Z1 1.5 min Z5 5 min Z1

RMI

CODE	DURATION	Z1	Z2	Z3	Z4	Z5	DESCRIPTION
RMI3	59	12	5	10	20	12	5 min Z1 5 min Z2 2 × (1 min Z5/2 min Z1) 2 × (3 min Z4/2 min Z1) 10 min Z3 2 min Z1 2 × (3 min Z4/2 min Z1) 2 × (1 min Z5/2 min Z1) 5 min Z1
RMI4	71	12	5	10	28	16	5 min Z1 5 min Z2 2 × (1.5 min Z5/2.5 min Z1) 2 × (5 min Z4/2 min Z1) 10 min Z3 2 min Z1 2 × (1.5 min Z5/2.5 min Z1) 2 × (5 min Z4/2 min Z1) 5 min Z1

Running Anaerobic Intervals (RAn)

Regular practice of the Running Anaerobic Intervals workout has the potential to transform your running through increased aerobic capacity and improved running economy. Best used in the early stages of a training cycle, this session serves as a springboard to better performance in more race-specific runs in the later stages, which in turn will deliver you to a strong closing leg on race day. Due to its prolonged and intense nature, the RAn should not be performed more often than once a week. Walking (rather than jogging) a portion of the rest interval is encouraged.

RAn

CODE	DURATION	Z1	Z2	Z3	Z4	Z5	DESCRIPTION
RAn1	60	50			10		15 min Z1 4 × (2.5 min Z4/5 min Z1) 15 min Z1
RAn2	60	47.5			12.5		15 min Z1 5 × (2.5 min Z4/5 min Z1) 7.5 min Z1
RAn3	60	45			15		15 min Z1 6 × (2.5 min Z4/5 min Z1)
RAn4	45	35			10		15 min Z1 4 × (2.5 min Z4/5 min Z1)
RAn5	44.5	37			7.5		15 min Z1 3 × (2.5 min Z4/5 min Z1) 7 min Z1

Running Short Intervals (RSI)

Unlike the very similar Running Hill Repeats workout, the Running Short Intervals workout is done on a flat surface, and as noted can be used in place of the RHR when no gradient can be found. Feel free to go hard.

RSI

CODE	DURATION	Z1	Z2	Z3	Z4	Z5	DESCRIPTION
RSI1	33	10	5			18	5 min Z1 5 min Z2 6 × (1 min Z5/2 min Z1) 5 min Z1
RSI2	39	10	5			24	5 min Z1 5 min Z2 8 × (1 min Z5/2 min Z1) 5 min Z1
RSI3	39	10	5			24	5 min Z1 5 min Z2 6 × (1.5 min Z5/2.5 min Z1) 5 min Z1
RSI4	45	10	5			30	5 min Z1 5 min Z2 10 × (1 min Z5/2 min Z1) 5 min Z1

Running Speed Play (RSP)

The Running Speed Play administers smaller doses of Zone 4 to provide a moderate stimulus for aerobic development without requiring you to go to the well. Because the rest intervals are short, you will likely pay a heavy price if you do the hard efforts too hard (in Zone 5).

RSP

CODE	DURATION	Z1	Z2	Z3	Z4	Z5	DESCRIPTION
RSP1	45	5	28		12		5 min Z1 28 min Z2 4 × (1 min Z4/2 min Z1)
RSP2	30	13	5		12		5 min Z1 5 min Z2 3 × (2 min Z4/2 min Z1) 8 min Z1
RSP3	30	10	5		15		5 min Z1 5 min Z2 5 × (1 min Z4/2 min Z1) 5 min Z1
RSP4	31	10	5		16		5 min Z1 5 min Z2 4 × (2 min Z4/2 min Z1) 5 min Z1
RSP5	33	10	5		18		5 min Z1 5 min Z2 6 × (1 min Z4/2 min Z1) 5 min Z1
RSP6	35	10	5		20		5 min Z1 5 min Z2 5 × (2 min Z4/2 min Z1) 5 min Z1

RSP

CODE	DURATION	Z1	Z2	Z3	Z4	Z5	DESCRIPTION
RSP7	36	10	5		21		5 min Z1 5 min Z2 7 × (1 min Z4/2 min Z1) 5 min Z1
RSP8	39	10	5		24		5 min Z1 5 min Z2 6 × (2 min Z4/2 min Z1) 5 min Z1
RSP9	39	10	5		24		5 min Z1 5 min Z2 8 × (1 min Z4/2 min Z1) 5 min Z1
RSP10	42	10	5		27		5 min Z1 5 min Z2 9 × (1 min Z4/2 min Z1) 5 min Z1
RSP11	43	10	5		28		5 min Z1 5 min Z2 7 × (2 min Z4/2 min Z1) 5 min Z1
RSP12	45	10	5		30		5 min Z1 5 min Z2 10 × (1 min Z4/2 min Z1) 5 min Z1
RSP13	47	10	5		32		5 min Z1 5 min Z2 8 × (2 min Z4/2 min Z1) 5 min Z1
RSP14	51	10	5		36		5 min Z1 5 min Z2 9 × (2 min Z4/2 min Z1) 5 min Z1

(continues)

(Running Speed Play continued)

RSP

CODE	DURATION	Z1	Z2	Z3	Z4	Z5	DESCRIPTION
RSP15	51	10	5		36		5 min Z1 5 min Z2 12 × (1 min Z4/2 min Z1) 5 min Z1
RSP16	51	10	20		21		5 min Z1 20 min Z2 7 × (1 min Z4/2 min Z1) 5 min Z1
RSP17	60	10	20		30		5 min Z1 20 min Z2 10 × (1 min Z4/2 min Z1) 5 min Z1
RSP18	48	10	10		28		5 min Z1 5 min Z2 7 × (2 min Z4/2 min Z1) 5 min Z2 5 min Z1
RSP19	49	10	15		24		5 min Z1 15 min Z2 8 × (1 min Z4/2 min Z1) 5 min Z1
RSP20	55	10	25		20		5 min Z1 15 min Z2 5 × (2 min Z4/2 min Z1) 10 min Z2 5 min Z1
RSP21	45	10	15		20		5 min Z1 10 min Z2 5 × (2 min Z4/2 min Z1) 10 min Z2 5 min Z1

Running Taper (RTa)

The Running Taper workout is intended to be used in race weeks, giving you just enough run intensity to stay sharp, but not so much as to burden you with fatigue. Cardiac lag will prevent your heart rate from reaching Zone 4 during these short intervals, so use perceived effort, power, or pace to regulate your intensity.

RTa

CODE	DURATION	Z1	Z2	Z3	Z4	Z5	DESCRIPTION
RTa1	10	5			6		5 min Z1, 6 × (20" Z4/40" rest)

ACKNOWLEDGMENTS

Like triathlon, book authorship is an individual sport in which success is impossible without the support of a team. Just as the triathlete depends on a coach, a bike mechanic, training partners, family, and others to achieve his or her goals, we have relied on a strong team of helpers serving a wide range of roles in our effort to create this book. In particular, we wish to acknowledge the invaluable contributions of Iris Bass, John Callos, Sarah Cotton, Betty Anne Crawford, Nataki Fitzgerald, Filip Galiza, AJ Gregg, Billy Hafferty, Stephen Kersh, Linda Konner, Bob Kusenberger, Fernanda Nunez, Leah Rosenfeld, Renée Sedliar, Stephen Seiler, Rebecca Warden, Danijela Vladimirov, and the good folks at Da Capo Lifelong Books.

INDEX

Index of Charts

ABOUT THE AUTHORS

MATT FITZGERALD is an acclaimed endurance sports coach, nutritionist, and author. His many previous books include *80/20 Running, How Bad Do You Want It?* and *The Endurance Diet*. Matt's byline has appeared in numerous major publications, including *Men's Health*, *Runner's World*, and *Triathlete*, and on such websites as Active.com and Triathlete.com. Certified by the International Society of Sports Nutrition, Matt developed the popular Diet Quality Score (DQS) smartphone app for nutrition tracking and provides individual nutritional counseling and coaching services through 8020endurance.com and mattfitzgerald.com. A runner since 1983 and a triathlete since 1998, Matt speaks frequently at conferences for endurance athletes all over the world.

DAVID WARDEN is an internationally recognized coach and author. His current and former clients include World Age Group Duathlon champions, Guinness World Record triathlon holders, and multiple full and 70.3 Ironman World Championship qualifiers. He is the coauthor of *Triathlon Science*, an industry standard text for triathlon coaches and academics. David's personal athletic resume consists of forty first-place overall wins in triathlon and duathlon, including the 2x USA Triathlon Rocky Mountain Region Sprint Triathlon Champion (2011, 2016). He has finished as the top American at the Mallora 70.3, Abu Dhabi International Half, and Balearic Olympic Championships. David offers endurance coaching and training plans at 8020endurance.com and dwcoaching.com.